HELENA TO VICKSBURG
A CIVIL WAR ODYSSEY

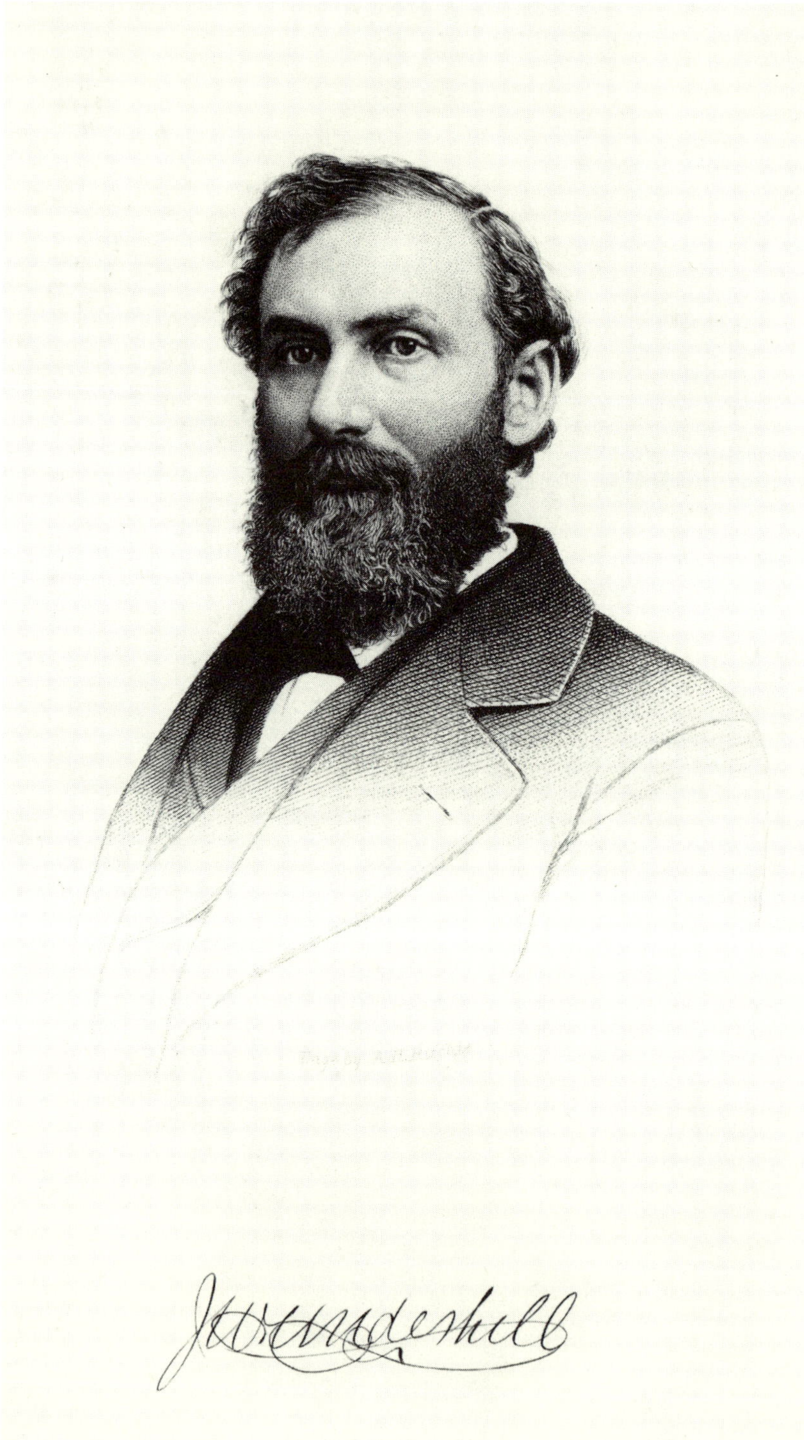

HELENA TO VICKSBURG
A CIVIL WAR ODYSSEY

The Personal Diary of
Joshua Whittington Underhill, Surgeon,
46th Regiment, Indiana Volunteer Infantry

23 October 1862 - 21 July 1863

EDITED BY
Christopher Morss

Heritage House, *Publishers*
LINCOLN CENTER, MASSACHUSETTS

For further information contact:

Heritage House, Publishers
25 Lincoln Road
P.O. Box 6135
Lincoln Center, Massachusetts 01773
(781) 259-8771

Book Design by Roger Gordy

ISBN 1-882063-49-X

Library of Congress Catalog Card Number: 99-75598
First Edition
Printed in the United States of America

Contents

Illustrations

PREFACE

Dr. Joshua Whittington Underhill's diary was missing for ten years until a Mr. C. G. Jennings of Delaware, Ohio very thoughtfully took the trouble to return it to him. In noting what had happened, Underhill made the most ironic comment in the diary: "Of course the memoranda are of no use to any one save myself."

No doubt other Civil War diaries are longer, more detailed, and more important, but all the same, Underhill was a perceptive and literate man some of whose observations and descriptions are superb. The family connection brings a special fascination to this diary, and certainly it is one more piece of the mosaic in reconstructing life during the Civil War.

Underhill married Eliza McPherson in 1874 and they had five children. Two girls died as small children and their son died in his twenties, but their daughters Nelle and Eliza lived to be ninety-nine and eighty-seven, respectively. Nelle was my grandmother, whom I knew well. Eliza, my great aunt, whom I knew but not as well, was the grandmother of Samuel B. Flora, Jr., my second cousin who eventually inherited the diary.

In mid-December, 1949, my parents and I flew from Boston to Los Angeles, in those days a fifteen hour trip by DC-4, with a stop in Cleveland and a plane change in Chicago – to attend the wedding of my older half brother, William Power Clancey, Jr., another great grandson of Dr. Underhill. We stayed with the younger surviving daughter of Dr. Underhill, Eliza Underhill Flora, then a matronly widow in her late sixties, who had a large, comfortable house in Pasadena at 1370 Ridge Avenue, close to the Huntington Hotel. I had not met Aunt Eliza before, and I found my great aunt a warm and outgoing person with a ready sense of humor. Also extending us a cordial welcome were her son, Sam, his wife, Dorothy, and their two sons, Neil and Sam, Jr., who at about fifteen and thirteen were wonderfully hospitable to their nine year old second cousin. They lived close by in San Marino. Probably

Aunt Eliza showed me her father's diary then, but she certainly did some fifteen years later, after she had moved to a bungalow at La Jolla, and awareness of its existence sat in my periphery.

Eventually the diary passed to her daughter, Jane Flora Ware, who gave it to her nephew Samuel B. Flora, Jr. He and I had spoken from time to time of "doing something" with the diary, but for some years we were both too busy with work to get around to it. However, an interest in getting it published did not go away, and by mid 1995, both of us had retired, and with time now to deal with the diary, Sam very generously agreed that I might borrow it. The weekend after Thanksgiving, 1995, I flew from Boston to St. Louis to collect it and spent several very happy days with Sam, his wife, Anne, and their grown daughter, Elizabeth.

The diary had been handsome when new. It had elegant paper marbled around the edges and an embossed red leather cover with a flap to hold it closed and a slot inside to hold a writing instrument. However, age had caused the binding to deteriorate. A cover had come off and a few pages were loose. Sam and I agreed that there was no point to commencing with preservation until I had finished my work.

After returning to Boston with the diary, I began transcribing it by hand, feeling that typing would be easier from my own transcription and less damaging to the book, since clearly, the book could not withstand complete photo copying. Initially, we had feared that some passages where the ink had faded would be unreadable, but with the aid of a magnifying glass and some educated guessing, it was possible to reconstruct the text, even though it did take a while to figure out Underhill's old-fashioned double "s" construction, which resembles an *f* and *s* together. He most likely used a steel pen, because the writing is distinctively heavy in some strokes and light in others, typical of such a nib. The ink is now a faded brown. Underhill's hand is firm, determined, and consistent, suggesting a decisive man of considerable intellect who could stand up for himself.

After the diary was copied longhand, it was transcribed onto the computer. As this job went along, several thoughts emerged. First, since the chief impetus was to get the diary published for the family, it seemed appropriate to add a section dealing both with biographical information about Dr. Underhill and some history of the family. As is so often true, one takes an interest in family history and genealogy only after those who could have answered many questions have left us. My grandmother, Nelle Underhill Green, Aunt Eliza's sister and the older surviving daughter of Dr. Underhill, I did know well, and it seemed important to write down the memories I can recall her recounting when I was quite young.

Second, while researchers having some interest in the diary would no doubt have considerable background information about the Civil War, the casual family reader might not – I certainly had forgotten all my high school history – and therefore it seemed appropriate to describe the context in which the entries are made. As well, references well understood by Dr. Underhill might not be understood today, and therefore a notes section seemed appropriate, especially since some are family references, which a researcher outside the family might not realize. The notes are arranged chronologically to match the diary entries.

Eventually, several sections emerged: the diary text itself, the annotations, and a background piece including some historical background as well as biographical and family history information. The original thought had been to separate the notes from the diary text itself, but as several readers reviewed the material, they commented that constant shifting between the text and the notes was irritating and disruptive. And yet, the thought of a page of text followed by footnotes in an academic format was forbidding, until Roger Gordy, a most talented designer, came up with the present format, which combines both the diary text and the notes in a pleasing manner, the diary text in large italics, the notes in plain style and a smaller font. This allows the reader interested only in the diary text to move on quickly. The background piece remains separate, and the later parts of it, especially, are unlikely to be of much interest to those outside the family.

Curiosity in the course of working with the diary has involved traveling to Cambridge, Fairview, and Cincinnati, Ohio; Indianapolis, Monticello and Burnettsville, Indiana; Memphis, Tennessee; Helena, Duvall's Bluff, St. Charles, and Clarendon, Arkansas; New Madrid, Missouri; Vicksburg, Mississippi and its environs; and to southern Maryland, where Underhill was born. To see "on the ground" where he lived and soldiered has been fascinating.

As the reader will see, the diary begins 23 October 1862 and ends 21 July 1863, when Underhill lost his diary. By pure luck it was found, and his having written his name and "Fairview, Guernsey County, Ohio," in the flyleaf enabled Mr. Jennings to return it to him. In the entry of 15 November 1873, the reader can experience Dr. Underhill's joy in having it back. Although his account of this is restrained, his pleasure is evident in his having turned the diary sideways to make this entry, his words tumbling down across six pages in a large and exuberant hand.

The period of his military service predated this diary and extended beyond it. Dr. Underhill numbered the pages from 1 to 239. He made entries on pages 1 to 111 from October 1862 until July 1863, and from 112 to 117 after he got the diary back in 1873, as well as recording mess bills, names of friends in other regiments, a poem, and river distances on pages 216-239. The diary is fascinating as is, but what an extensive account he would have left us had the empty pages he numbered been filled up!

Sherborn, Massachusetts
September 1999

ACKNOWLEDGMENTS

One hero of this story is the late C. G. Jennings, of Delaware, Ohio. When he came upon Dr. Underhill's diary among the effects of a relative who was a Vicksburg veteran, he went to considerable trouble to locate Dr. Underhill and return the diary to him. Had he not been so gracious, we would not have the diary today. Our thanks must be posthumous.

Without the help of a great many people, much of the information in this book would not have been available. Bruce Johnson, Eric Mundell, Peter T. Harstad, and Leigh Darbee at the Indiana Historical Society have offered kind assistance. Larry Liggett and Joseph Reinhart provided information about Camp Wickliffe. Michael Flannery at the Lloyd Library in Cincinnati has responded graciously to requests for information, as has Margaret Meade, at Spring Grove Cemetery. Judy Beland and Lucretia McClure arranged for a visit to Harvard's Countway Library, and Mary Kestle and Joyce Sharp, of the Monticello-Union Township Public Library in Monticello, Indiana, went far out of their way to dig up information and to make a visit to that library profitable. Fr. Jerry Gardner at St. Patrick Church, Fayetteville, Ohio, researched the church records for Underhill material, while Barbara Van Brimmer, at Ohio State University, pored through archives for information about J. T. McPherson. Melissa McDermott generously gave her time to search the Marietta College records, as did Robin Hanson at Muskingum College. David Pittinger of the Recorder's Office in Cincinnati spent an inordinate amount of time helping to track down deeds. He is truly a public servant. Nancy Eckerman at the Ruth Lilly Medical Library at Indiana University searched valiantly for information on Underhill's classmate, William Fleming. Evelyn Griffin and other staff members at the Phillips County Museum and Library in Helena, Arkansas were most kind and welcoming. Jennifer Small, Barbara Wiley, and Joanne McCarten at the Emma Willard School extended themselves to provide information from the school's archives.

Henry Hicks at the Needham, Massachusetts Historical Society took precious time to review the diary and background material and to offer valuable comments.

Melissa Essex and her predecessor, Richard Goodwin, keepers of the Finley Room at the Guernsey County Public Library in Cambridge, Ohio, have been infinitely helpful, both through the mail and on-scene. Melissa has many times sent on information she has found that she felt might be germane, and I am much indebted.

Despite heavy demands as Director of the Edward H. Nabb Research Center for Delmarva History and Culture in Salisbury, Maryland, Rebecca Miller has been most generous with assistance, both at the Center and with e-mail, as has been her associate, Corinne Les Callette.

At the Cincinnati Historical Society, Bill Graver helped to track down deeds. Anne B. Shepherd and other staff members, especially Chris Bell-Puckett, have answered numerous letters and questions and fetched countless books. I am grateful to them for their generous and unstinting help.

I am indebted to Dr. Arthur G. King of Cincinnati for his encouragement, candid guidance, and for generously allowing the use of his material. A medical historian, he alone has kept Dr. Underhill's accomplishments alive.

I offer profound thanks to Billie Broaddus, Director of the Medical Heritage Center at the University of Cincinnati. Gracious, welcoming, and ever imaginative about what source to consult next, Billie has answered endless e-mail messages requesting information and has made several visits to the Center most worthwhile. Without her generous help, none of the medical history in this volume would have been available.

The book would never have taken shape without the experienced guidance and editorial expertise of Mary Ann Hales at Heritage House, Publishers. Her encouragement and tactful manner have made suggested revisions welcome. I am deeply grateful to her and to her associates, John

C. MacLean and Roger Gordy. Besides writing many of the picture captions, John has offered valuable criticism and challenged several assertions which warranted revisiting. Roger has produced a most gratifying book design. Will Williamson's enthusiasm in photographing some of the diary pages and then scanning the slides has been infectious.

And finally, I am most grateful to my cousins, Sam and Anne Flora. Anne took on the enormous task of being an editor and critic, and her suggestions have been immensely valuable. Both she and Sam have offered hospitality, encouragement and sound advice, and without Sam's great generosity in allowing me to borrow Dr. Underhill's diary in the first place, this volume would not have appeared.

HELENA TO VICKSBURG
A CIVIL WAR ODYSSEY

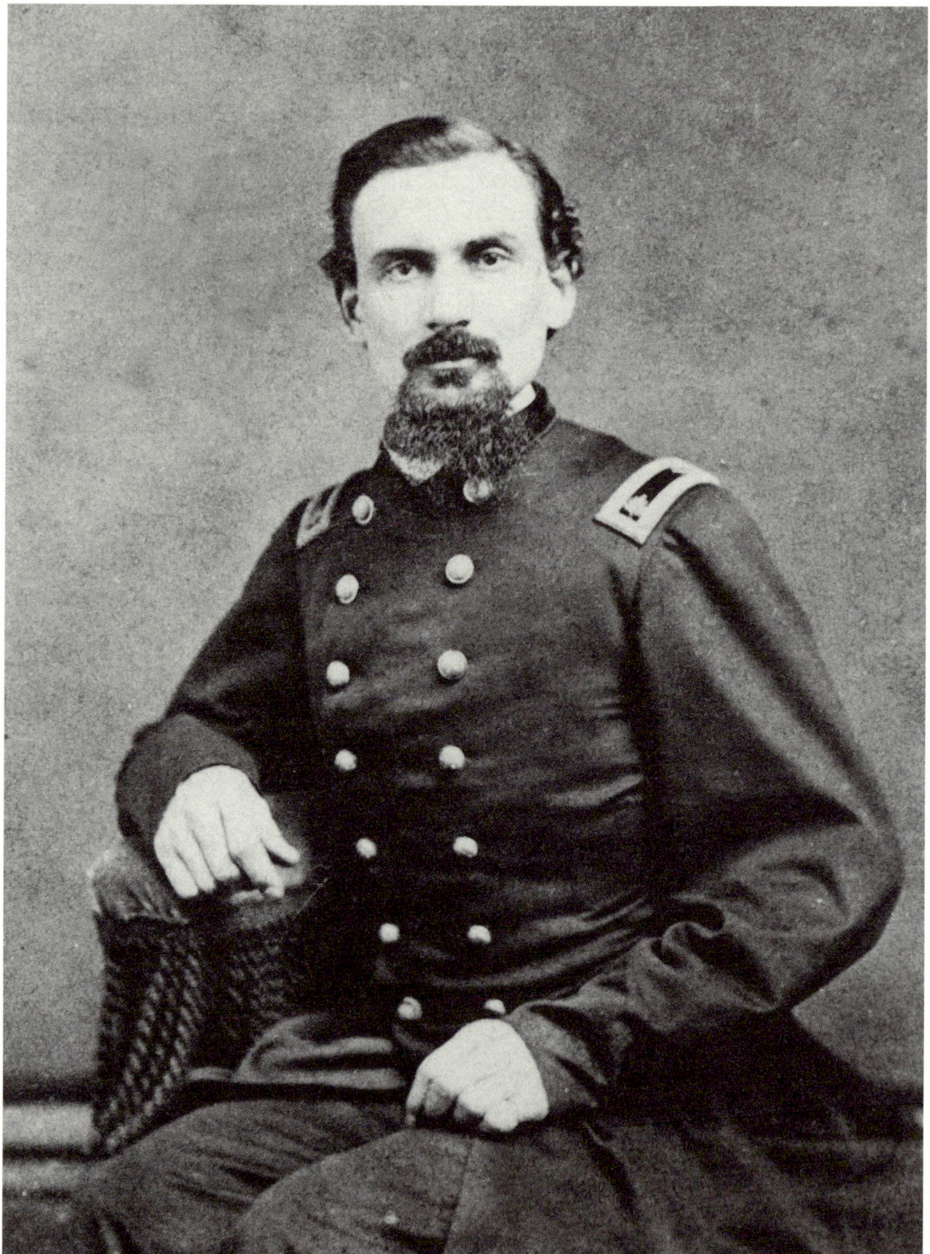

Joshua Whittington Underhill
46th Regiment, Indiana Volunteer Infantry
Photograph taken at Lexington, KY, 1864.

Memoranda.

Memoranda

Helena, Ark's. Oct. 23rd, 1862

Pleasant day. Weather been mild for the last two weeks when we had a sudden cold change. Yesterday a party of 200 guirrellas attacked and captured a number of teams that were out foraging—70 guards quite a number of teamsters captured. Wrote a letter to Robt. McMillen of Logansport concerning death of his son.

NOTES FOR October 23

Helena, Ark's: Helena, Phillips County, Arkansas, lies on the west bank of the Mississippi River about sixty miles south of Memphis and forty-five miles north of the mouth of the White River. In the 1860 census, Phillips County had 8817 slaves, 3558 adult white males and 2465 adult white females. That part of the town for perhaps half a mile inland from the Mississippi was essentially flat and at the time of the Civil War extended back from the river six blocks and was eight blocks long. Behind the town lie steep ridges, part of what is called Crowley's Ridge. Helena was a substantial town where Underhill bought his diary book and an important river port where mule trains would bring cotton for shipment to New Orleans. After Union General Samuel R. Curtis occupied Helena late in June 1862, it became an important staging base and supply depot for the Vicksburg Campaign. The Indiana 46th was based in Helena from 15 July 1862 until 11 April 1863, when it left for Vicksburg. The riverfront today has changed greatly, since a big levee has been constructed along the river bank, making the river invisible from the town.

Son of Robt. McMillen: Adams McMillen, Pvt., Co. B. Residence: Logansport, Indiana. Date of muster 5 November 1861. Died at Memphis, 14 July 1862. His cause of death is shown neither in the Indiana Adjutant General's Report nor in the *History of the Forty-Sixth Regiment Indiana Volunteer Infantry*.

Oct. 24.

Yesterday our cavalry scoured the country for miles back of town but ascertained little as to the capturing of our teams. They brought in a few prisoners burned several houses and devastated plantations. The officer who had charge of the expedition has been arrested for such wholesale savages. Rec'd "Jeffersonian" containing my last communication – it has been so mutilated that I cannot think I will write another for the paper. Rec'd. also a no. of "Monticello Herald"– wrote private letter to Ed. of "Jeffersonian."

NOTES FOR October 24
The "Jeffersonian": The *Jeffersonian* was and remains a newspaper published in Cambridge, Guernsey County, Ohio. Underhill had grown up in Fairview, Ohio, a small town about fifteen miles east of Cambridge with an 1860 population of 365. Since Fairview was too small to support a paper, he subscribed to the Cambridge one. No copy of the issue referred to could be obtained to read what Underhill had written.

The "Monticello Herald": For three months before enlisting, Underhill had been living about seventy-five miles north-northwest of Indianapolis in Burnettsville, White County, Indiana, having moved from Fairview, Ohio. The *Monticello Herald* was published at Monticello, Indiana, a town about eight miles west of Burnettsville with an 1860 population of about 1800 and the seat of White County.

Helena, Ark's.
Oct. 25th

Quite a sudden change occurred in the weather last night. To-day it is snowing a little.

Oct. 26.

Last night water froze ½ inch thick – Towards noon to-day it became much more pleasant.

Oct. 27.

Yesterday evening two of our boys while on picket across the river were shot. Mart Rutter Co: A killed and Daniel Samsel Co B. severely wounded. Two of the 43rd Ind. were also killed and two wounded.

NOTES FOR October 27

Mart Rutter: Martin L. Rutter, Pvt., Co. A. Residence: Pittsburg, Indiana. Killed by guerrillas near Helena, Arkansas, 26 October 1862.

Daniel Samsel: Daniel W. Samsel, Pvt., Co. D. Residence: Logansport, Indiana. Date of muster: 5 November 1861. Shown in the *History of the Forty-Sixth Regiment Indiana Volunteer Infantry* as David. The Adjutant General's Report lists him as Daniel and Underhill's rendering as Daniel is very clear. Discharged 8 February 1863 because of disability.

Helena, Ark's.
Oct. 29, 1862

This evening the 26th Iowa came down the river also reenforced by the 24th Iowa two days ago. It is rumored that 10,000 new troops will soon arrive. A little steamer, "The Little Rock," with 100 prisoners came up under flag of truce. A portion of the prisoners were those captured a few days since while out with the teams foraging.

NOTES FOR October 29
Little Rock: a stern-wheel packet built at Cincinnati in 1858 and enrolled at New Orleans in January 1859.[1]

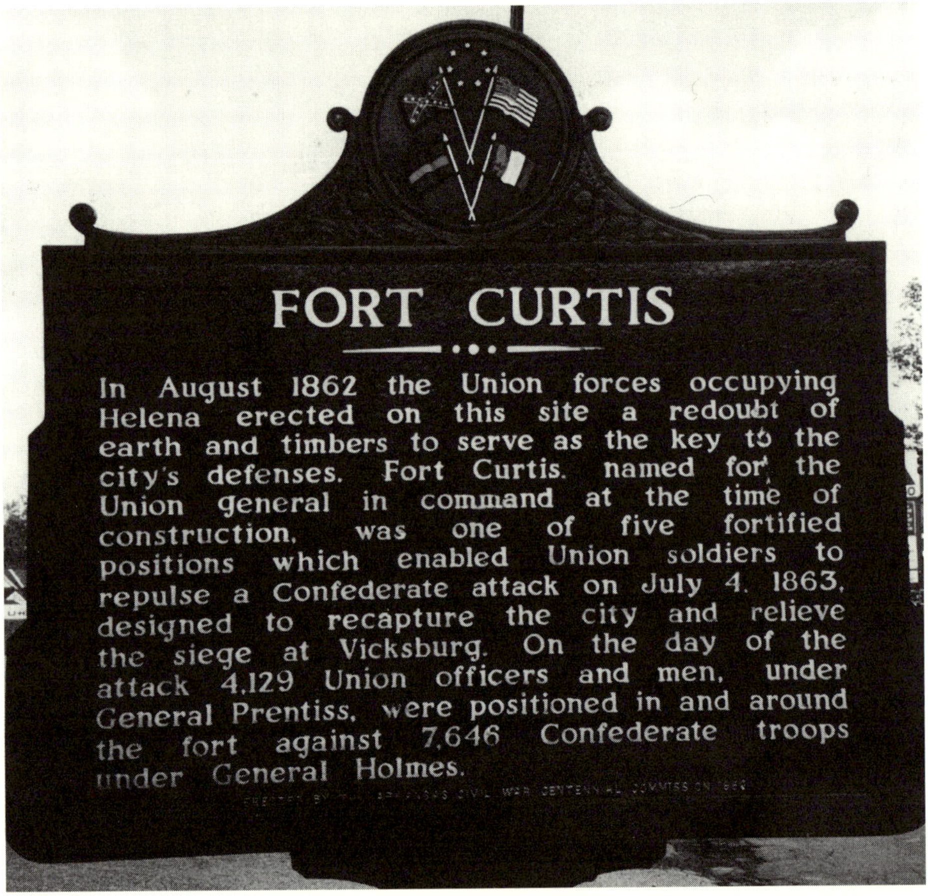

Historical marker, Perry Street, Helena, Arkansas.

Oct. 30

Fort dedicated. Salutes fired from fort replied to by the fleet and surrounding batteries. Infantry went through all evolutions of field practice. Fort christened "Fort Curtis."

NOTES FOR October 30
Fort Curtis: Fort Curtis was named after (Union) Major General Samuel R. Curtis (1807-1866). In the spring of 1862, Curtis had been commander of the Union troops in Arkansas. His objective was Little Rock, but since other Union forces were drained off by operations in Tennessee and could not support him, he had had to withdraw. He abandoned Batesville, Arkansas, on June 24 and moved his troops southeast to Helena, where in late June, they established the base where Underhill's diary opens. In July 1863, some weeks after the Indiana 46th had left, Confederate troops under Lieutenant General Theophilus Holmes attacked the fort, then numbering about 4000 men, in an attempt to distract Union forces from their campaign against Vicksburg. We might infer from the diary that on occasion when Underhill was there, Fort Curtis and Helena comprised considerably more than four thousand troops. The fort itself covered a city block. In September of 1862, General Curtis was assigned to the command of the Department of the Missouri and was relieved by Brigadier General Frederick Steele. Major General B. M. Prentiss then relieved Steele and was commander at the time of the July 1863 attack. Underhill describes Prentiss in detail in a 15 March 1863 entry. No traces of Fort Curtis remain in Helena today except for an historical marker on Perry Street showing where it stood, six or seven blocks back from the river.

Underhill's regiment never camped within the fort, and Underhill did not go inside it until November 23. In early August, for example, the regiment was encamped a few miles south of Helena at the Pillow Farm, and from time to time Underhill notes campsite changes.

Nov. 4

Last few days fine weather. Rec'd and answered Dr. Washburne's letter, also rec'd letter from Lina. Wrote G. W. Spencer few days since.

NOTES FOR November 4

Dr. Washburne: Israel B. Washburn. Residence: Logansport, Indiana. Date of muster: 2 December 1861. He was a corporal in Company I but was promoted to assistant surgeon 27 December 1862 and to surgeon 17 October 1863. He mustered out when his term expired 28 December 1864 and was replaced by Underhill.

Lina: Lina's identity is a mystery. She appears in entries of November 4, November 6, and November 22, but not again. On December 29 is the first reference to "Linnie," later referred to rather coyly as Linnie J., whose identity also is a mystery, although by the frequency of the references to her, it sounds as if she and Underhill might have been sweethearts. It appears unlikely that Lina and Linnie are the same person.

G. W. Spencer: George W. Spencer, 1st Lt., Co. E. Residence: Monticello, Indiana. Enlisted 5 November 1861; commissioned first lieutenant 12 June 1862. Honorably discharged 7 June 1863. He was a nephew of Dr. Robert Spencer and a first cousin of Dr. William Spencer. In an 1881 postscript penciled in his diary at the back, Underhill records Spencer's "terrible death by poisoning" some years after the war. According to a local newspaper account, Spencer had returned from Chicago feeling deeply fatigued, and sensing illness coming on, had taken what he thought was a dose of quinine. He took instead corrosive sublimate, a highly potent poison kept by farmers to rid farm animals of vermin. He endured several days of torture before dying at 11 PM on Monday, 7 August 1876.

Helena Ark's.
Nov. 6, 1862

Yesterday wrote a letter to Lina. To-day one home. Reg't, (30th Iowa), came down. Yesterday came 29th Wisconsin. All new reg'ts.

NOTES FOR November 6

home: Since being essentially orphaned as a small boy, Underhill had lived with John and Eleanor (Elenor) (Nellie) Gilbert since

1840 and is shown in the census by name as living with them in Fairview, Ohio, at ages 13 in 1850 and as a doctor at age 23, in 1860. They had also taken in as a young orphan her nephew, J. T. McPherson (1824-1894), who became Underhill's medical preceptor. (For *preceptor*, see note for 15 November 1873.) The Gilberts had no children. John's dates are 1803-1882, Eleanor's 1797-1872. John appears to have remarried, since in his will he mentions a wife Elizabeth but also a first wife. Although Underhill never mentions the Gilberts by name, it seems safe to assume that the Gilberts are "home." The Gilberts are buried in the Fairview Cemetery.

November 10

Last night I attended church in town at the Episcopalian. Rev. Sawyer Chaplain of 47th Ind preached. First sermon I have heard for one year. Rec'd letter from Newell Kennon which I do not think I will answer. Sent two papers to Lina and wrote a letter home.

NOTES FOR November 10

the Episcopalian: St. John's Episcopal Church, established in 1853. The present church stands at the corner of Perry and Pecan Streets. It was built in 1914 after a fire destroyed an older building on the site. However, the church to which Underhill refers predates these and stood on the southwest corner of Cherry and Rightor Streets. Completed in 1861, it was small, made of cyprus, and was confiscated for Federal use during the Civil War. The church was later sold and no longer stands but appears in an extant photograph. Episcopal Bishop and later Confederate General Leonidas Polk had arrived in Helena in 1839 to hold what was perhaps the first Episcopal service in Arkansas. The present church is a mere block away from where Fort Curtis stood, whereas the original church was several blocks away.

Rev. Sawyer: Samuel W. Sawyer. Residence: Marion, Indiana. Date of commission: 10 October 1861. Date of muster:

13 December 1861. Chaplain of the 47th Indiana. Resigned 9 October 1864.

Newell Kennon: The Kennons in Guernsey and Belmont counties in Ohio were prolific, and several men in the family were called Newell. Most likely Underhill is referring to the Hon. Newell Kennon. Born in 1810, he was a younger brother of Nancy (Kennon) Gilliland and uncle of Mary (Gilliland) McPherson, Underhill's preceptor's wife. Kennon served as a justice of the peace, a state legislator, postmaster in Fairview, and during the administration of Franklin Pierce, was appointed to an important post in the Treasury Department in Washington which he held for twenty years. In 1880 he ran for Probate Judge and won, despite being a Democrat in a strongly Republican area. He outlived his wife and four children and died in 1883. He is buried in the cemetery in Fairview, Ohio.

However, Underhill could also be referring to Newell W. Kennon (1830-1883), son of John and Elizabeth (Giffee), listed in the 1860 census as a physician; or to Newell G. Kennon (1841-1863), son of James and Rose (Kennon).

Nov. 11

Yesterday the Lieut. Col. and major of the 26th Iowa were captured while out a short distance beyond pickets. Quite a joke on the new Reg'ts.

Helena, Ark's.
Nov. 12, 1862

Yesterday and to-day have been very rainy days. First rain for several weeks. It is rumored that recruiting has commenced here for the Regular Service.

Nov. 13

Twenty-fifth Iowa arrived.

Nov. 16

This (Sunday) morning an expedition started for some point unknown down the Mississippi. Gen. Hovey's division about 7,000 troops under command of Gen. Washburn 14 steamers laden with troops. Took rations for 10 days and expect to return. No one allowed to pass pickets since order for expedition was given. I am left in charge of 35 sick the hospital portion of which will be seen by Dr. Lyons of 24th Iowa. Rec'd letter from Sullie. Mail boat (Eugene) had sunk and mail remained under water three days.

NOTES FOR November 16

Gen. Hovey: (Union) Brigadier General Alvin Peterson Hovey (1821-1891) was Underhill's division commander and an Indiana lawyer and politician. He served in the Mexican War and lost a bid for Congress in 1858. He was in McClernand's corps at Vicksburg, where a bust of him stands in the Military Park. Grant praised him for action at Champion Hill. After the war he served in Peru as a diplomat, served two terms as a congressman and died in office while governor of Indiana.[2]

Gen. Washburn: (Union) Major General Cadwallader Coldon Washburn, 1818-1882. A Maine native, he was a businessman and lawyer in Wisconsin before becoming a Republican congressman in 1854. Some documents spell his last name *Washburn* and others *Washburne.* Dr. Underhill usually used *Washburn.* The General appears to have spelled his name as *Washburn* while his Illinois Congressman brother, Elihu, spelled his name as *Washburne.* He commanded the cavalry in Curtis's army in Arkansas and later commanded several divisions at Vicksburg. After the war he resumed his political career and later made a fortune in what was to become General Mills.[3]

Dr. Lyons: Henry M. Lyons, Assistant Surgeon, 24th Iowa

Infantry. Residence: Cedar Rapids. Born in New York. Date of commission: 22 September 1862.

Sullie: Sullie's identity is unknown.

Eugene: a side-wheel packet built at Parkersburg, Virginia in 1860. She was under charter when she hit the wreck of another vessel at Osceola, Arkansas, 14 November 1862, with the loss of life estimated at fifteen.[4]

Helena Ark's.
Nov. 18

Weather cloudy and rainy last two days. Getting along well with sick, little lonesome since regiment has left. Rec'd letter to-day from Celia – quite refreshing and served to dispel a cloud of the blues. Also rec'd "Monticello Herald." A few days since wrote home.

NOTES FOR November 18

Celia: Celia's identity is not known. On November 18, he writes of having received a letter from her which dispelled "the blues." On November 25 he writes back to her and only then on December 31, notes receiving a letter from her that she is married and living in Allegheny City, Tennessee. One could surmise she was a girl he was fond of, perhaps someone he had known at Madison College.

Nov. 20

Last night returned the "Gladiator" from the expedition. Came for 10 days more provisions. Reports leaving the fleet at the mouth of White River. Rumored that Steele's and Osterhaus' divisions are en route for this point via the Mississippi River. Not having found the enemy they returned from Pilot Knob, Mo. to St. Louis where they embarked. Arrived two new regts. (Iowa 28th and 31st). River very low. Weather more pleasant today.

NOTES FOR November 20

The *Gladiator*: a side-wheel packet built at Belle Vernon, Pennsylvania and completed at Pittsburgh in 1857. It had seen service in the Tennessee River campaign.[5]

White River: The White River runs roughly south through Arkansas and drains into the Mississippi about forty-five miles south of Helena. It was navigable by steamboat for a considerable distance upstream but only if there were enough water.

Gen. Steele: (Union) Brigadier General Frederick Steele (1819-1868) relieved General Curtis as commander of Fort Curtis at Helena. Later, as a major general, he commanded a division under General Sherman at Vicksburg. He took part in the Chickasaw Bayou attack and in numerous other engagements.

Gen. Osterhaus: (Union) Brigadier General Peter J. Osterhaus (1823-1917) was a Prussian born in Koblenz who left Europe after 1848. He proved a very successful general. Besides other engagements, he was at the battle for Port Gibson and commanded a division under McClernand at Vicksburg.

Nov. 22nd

Last night expedition returned. Their destination was Arkansas Post on the Arkansas River about 8 miles from its mouth. The intention was to proceed up White River a short distance perhaps to Prairie Landing and from thence march across to the Post. The White was found too low to allow the passage of the boats. Owing to the swamps with which the country abounds about the mouth of the White it was impossible to make the march from that point or from the mouth of the Arkansas. Therefore after making every reasonable attempt it was found impossible to proceed and the expedition was compelled to return. It has been ascertained that Arkansas Post has been pretty well fortified and is garrisoned by 5,000 Secesh. They therefore have command of the Arkansas at that point. Whether another attempt will be made to dislodge them is not yet certain. Gen. Steele and Osterhaus are returning. Their advance came in by the river this afternoon. New Iowa Reg't (43rd) arrived last night.

Rec'd letter from Lina, also from Isaac Lankford and the Jeffersonian. Wrote to Celia.

NOTES FOR November 22

Arkansas Post: Arkansas Post was one of the earliest European communities in the lower Mississippi Valley, having been settled in 1686. Its population was greatest when it was the capital of Arkansas but declined after the capital was moved to Little Rock in 1821. It lies on the north side of the Arkansas River, which at that point flows roughly southeast through Arkansas to drain forty miles beyond into the Mississippi. Fort Hindman at Arkansas Post was held by five thousand men under the Confederate Brigadier General T. J. Churchill until its capture by Major General John A. McClernand in January 1863.

Prairie Landing: Prairie Landing, Arkansas was about twenty-two miles upstream from the mouth of the White River.

Secesh: Secesh is a colloquial term for the Secessionists.

Isaac Lankford: Possibly Isaac Smith Lankford, b. 1814; d. 1882, son of Henry Lankford; m. Sarah A. Coulbourn. Lankford is an old Quindocqua, Maryland name, and Underhill's great grandmother on his mother's side was Isabella Lankford. Somerset County, Maryland marriage records list several Isaac Lankfords. It has not been possible to identify this particular Isaac Lankford, although it is quite likely he lived in the Quindocqua area and was a distant cousin.

Nov. 23rd. Sunday Night

Just returned from church – heard Rev. Sawyer chaplain of 47th Ind. preach text 1st chap and 21st verse of 1st Corinthians. He is a minister in Methodist church. Service held in Episcopal church. Today I was in the interior of Fort Curtis for the first time. It is a pretty substantial fortification of large guns, largest 42 pounder, two small pieces – batteries will be planted on surrounding hills. Its size is just one city square. Weather still pleasant and mild.

Nov. 25th

Several new recruits arrived to day, also recruiters. Rumors are to day that another expedition leaves down the river with 20 days' rations to morrow. Rec'd. letter from Dr. McPherson giving sad intelligence of deaths of Dr. Withney Kennon and Wm. Tillet. The former died of congestive chills latter of Camp Fever.

NOTES FOR November 25

Dr. McPherson: Jeremiah Townsend McPherson, 1824-1894. Dr. McPherson was Underhill's medical preceptor and later his father-in-law. He married Mary Wilson Gilliland April 25, 1848. They had three children: Eliza "Lida," who married Underhill; Mary Kennon McPherson, who married William Henry Dunham; and Jennie Crew McPherson, who married John Ogier. Dr. McPherson practiced for some years in Fairview, Guernsey County, Ohio. In 1876, he moved to Cambridge, the seat for Guernsey County, where he lived until his death.

Dr. Withney Kennon: b. 1829, d. 1 November 1862. He was a first cousin of Mary (Gilliland) McPherson, the wife of Underhill's preceptor. Withney's parents were Margaret and Abner Kennon, Abner being a brother of Nancy (Kennon) Gilliland, Mary (Gilliland) McPherson's mother. In the 1850 Belmont County census, Withney is shown as Whitney, but Abner's mother was Elizabeth Withney and the census taker misspelled his name. At that time he was age 22, a farmer living with his parents. By June of 1860, he was still single, 31, a physician, living at the American House Hotel in Beverly, Ohio, in the northwest corner of Washington County, his personal estate valued at $3000. Congestive chills are pernicious malaria with gastrointestinal congestion and diarrhea, preceded by a chill. He is buried in the cemetery at Fairview, Ohio as is his younger brother Milton, who also became a doctor, practicing in Barnesville, Belmont County, Ohio, where he died in 1921.

Wm. Tillet: Most likely William Tillet listed in the 1860 Fairview census as age 14, the son of James Tillet, 58, a tailor, and his wife Uree, 52. At the time of his death he would have been

16 or 17. Since the news of his death came from Dr. McPherson, then in Fairview, it would appear that he died in Fairview, since he would have been very young for the army, although the Tillets had an older son, Ignatius, who appears in Underhill's list at the end of the diary as a member of Company A in the Ohio 25th. Camp fever is another name for typhus.

Nov. 27th

The rumored expedition left this afternoon but to what point is not known. They went down the river. The force consisted of perhaps ten thousand Infantry, Cavalry, and Artillery. The last expedition instead of being commanded by Washburn was under Gen. Hovey. To-day is Thanksgiving Day. Wrote a letter home. Weather clear and cool.

December 1st, 1862

Last night had a heavy thunder storm. Warm and pleasant to day. Rec'd letter from home. Three boat-loads of Secesh prisoners arrived. Eucre party to night.

NOTES FOR December 1
eucre: euchre, a popular nineteenth century card game.

Dec. 5th

This morning opened up with blistering weather. Snow fell towards noon. Sun broke out and to night weather is quite moderate. Last night arrived Dr. Washburn from home. Saw Sam Keller who was discharged recently from Memphis. Rumors rec'd that some cavalry of the expedition that left on the 27th ult. had a skirmish also that at another time our boys captured a number of cars and cannon and tore up the R.R. from Grenada to Memphis. Rumored, too, that they will return in a few days.

NOTES FOR December 5
Sam Keller: Samuel Keller, Pvt., Co. F. Residence: Delphi, Indiana. Date of muster 14 November 1861. Discharged at Memphis because of disability 13 November 1862.

ult.: short for ultimo, meaning the month previous.

Grenada: a town in Mississippi approximately seventy miles southeast of Helena, Arkansas.

Dec. 7th

Expedition returned to day Sunday. They proceeded across the R.R. from Grenada to Memphis, to the Ohio and Mississippi R.R. both of which roads they destroyed for some distance, burning several important bridges and destroying the tracks for some distance. Thus Price's communication to the rear is cut off. The expedition having accomplished the object for which it was sent out returned to day having lost a few men by bushwhacking. A few prisoners were brought in. Our cavalry were within five miles of Grenada.

Wrote a short letter home.

NOTES FOR December 7
Price: Sterling Price (1809-1867) was a Confederate major general. Virginia born, he moved to Missouri, serving as a state legislator, governor, and representative in Congress. He fought in the Mexican War and joined the Confederacy in 1861, spending much of the war trying to get Missouri for the Confederacy.

bushwhacking: guerrilla warfare

Helena
Dec. 11th

Fine weather for the last week. Few days since sent away 16 sick to Gen. Hospital. Yesterday resigned Dr. Haymond first asst. surgeon of our regiment. Second asst. Dr. Spencer reported absent without leave. Resigned also Capt. Cowden and Lieut. Benner (as G & G). Wrote a letter to Jno. Dixon.

To-morrow will be one year since we left Camp Logan, Logansport Ind.
Poker party tonight. Players Lt. Fisher, Orderly P. M. Meek, C. J. Armstrong and myself.

NOTES FOR December 11
Dr. Haymond: William S. Haymond, Assistant Surgeon. Residence: Monticello, Indiana. Date of commission: 19 November 1861. Date of muster: 20 November 1861. Resigned 29 December 1862. He was a graduate of the Bellevue Hospital Medical College in New York as well as a talented mathematician and linguist. After the war he served in the U.S. House of Representatives.

Dr. Spencer: William Spencer, Assistant Surgeon, 46th Indiana. Residence: Monticello, Indiana. Commissioned as Captain, Co. E, 4 October 1861. Date of commission and muster as assistant surgeon: 7 July 1862. Resigned 29 December 1862. While Dr. Underhill notes his resignation on December 14 "a few days since," it may be that the official date of resignation is December 29. Spencer then became Assistant Surgeon of the Indiana 73rd, the same unit in which his father, Dr. Robert Spencer, was serving. He was captured in Alabama in April 1863 and was held until November 1864. He then served with the 10th Tennessee Cavalry and later as a staff officer. After the war he returned to Monticello. Before the war, both he and his father had been professors at the Cincinnati College of Medicine and Surgery, where Underhill had known them, and as Captain Spencer he enlisted Underhill in the 46th. He married Harriett V. Kistler in 1856. They had three children. She died in 1888 and he died in Monticello in 1901.

Capt. Cowden: Shown in the Indiana Adjutant General's report as Captain Joseph D. Cowdin, Company G. Residence: Monticello, Indiana. Date of commission as first lieutenant: 4 October 1861. Date of commission and muster as captain: 17 November 1862. Resigned 23 December 1862. The 1860 White County census shows him as age 31 and the county auditor. He assumed this post first in 1853 and again in 1856, after his successor died in office.

Lt. Benner: Joseph H. Benner, 2nd Lt., Co. I. Residence:

Lagro, Indiana. Enlisted as sergeant 2 December 1861. Date of commission and muster as second lieutenant: 22 May 1862. Resigned 29 December 1862.

Jno.: An abbreviation for "John." John Dixon appears in the 1860 White County census as a resident of Burnettsville, age 27, a journeyman carpenter born in Kentucky and married to Eliza, 34, born in Pennsylvania, with a son Wilson, age 1.

Lt. Fisher: Charles F. Fisher, Sgt., Co. E. Residence: Battle Ground, Indiana. Enlisted 5 November 1861. Date of commission and muster as second lieutenant: 12 June 1862. Date of muster as first lieutenant: 6 August 1863. Promoted to Captain. Date of commission: 27 December 1864. Date of muster: 19 January 1865. Mustered out with the regiment.

Orderly P. M. Meek: Preston Meek, Sgt., Co. E. Enlisted 5 November 1861. Commissioned second lieutenant 1 July 1863. Meek mustered out with the regiment as a sergeant and not as a lieutenant because the company was below minimum. He is shown in the *History of the Forty-Sixth Regiment Indiana Volunteer Infantry* as Preston S. Meek, while Underhill shows him as P. M. Meek. The 1860 White County, Indiana census shows a Preston Meek, age 19, farm laborer, son of Richard, 42, and Ellen 42, with numerous siblings, living in Burnettsville.

C. J. Armstrong: Clinton J. Armstrong, Cpl., Co. E. Residence: Delphi, Indiana. Date of muster: 5 November 1861. Died at Helena, 2 February 1863. See diary entry of February 4.

Helena, Arkansas
Dec. 14 Sunday Night

Last two days been quite warm, too warm to be comfortable with a blouse. Rained a little yesterday and this morning. Today preached Chaplain Robb of our reg't. his first discourse, only came to reg't ten days since. Heard Chaplain Filet preach to night in the Episcopalian church in town. Quite an able discourse. Text Malachi: Chap. 1. verse 6. followed by a sort of general Class meeting. Two nights since began medical quiz. Members Drs.

Coleman, Culberson Asst. of 43rd Ind. Washburne and myself – meet every night and discuss a particular subject. Dr. W. S. Spencer resigned a few days since and hence will not be mustered out as before stated.

NOTES FOR December 14
Chaplain Robb: The Reverend Hamilton Robb. Residence: Delphi, Indiana. Date of commission: 16 December 1862. Date of muster: 10 January 1863. In the late 1830's, he had been pastor of a Methodist-Episcopal church in Guernsey County, Ohio, as well as the county treasurer. Although Underhill spent most of his youth in Guernsey County, it is highly unlikely that the two met then. The census of 1850 for Clark County, Indiana, lists him in Jeffersonville as a Baptist clergyman, age 49, with his wife, Sarah, age 44, two daughters, 14 and 12, and a son, 9. He was elected chaplain 5 November 1862, Robert Irvin having resigned in May 1862. Robb was beloved by the regiment. He was taken prisoner at the battle of the Sabine Crossroads. According to the *History of the Forty-Sixth Regiment Indiana Volunteer Infantry*, he was seventy years old at the time, but if his age in the 1850 census was correct, he would have been closer to sixty-five. He mustered out with the regiment.

Dr. Coleman: Horace Coleman, Surgeon, 46th Indiana. Residence: Logansport, Indiana. Date of muster: 30 September 1861. Date of commission: 7 October 1861. Resigned 31 July 1863.

Culberson: David P. Culbertson, Assistant Surgeon, 43rd Indiana. Residence: Edwardsport, Indiana. Date of commission: 23 September 1862. Date of muster: 3 October 1862. Resigned 9 April 1864.

Dr. W. S. Spencer: He was William G. Spencer.

Helena, Ark's.
December 17th

Pleasant day. Night of 14th heavy storm. Stormed all next day. Yesterday sent joint recommendation to Gov. Morton for the appointment of Dr.

Washburn and myself to fill the two vacancies which will undoubtedly be made vacant by the resignations of Drs. Haymond and Spencer. Recommend got up by Col. Bringhurst and surgeon also separate recommend signed by Dr. Jessup senior surgeon division and Dr. Castlebury and Dr. Haymond. Wrote a letter to George W. Spencer. News came of death of Reese Laird.

NOTES FOR December 17

Gov. Morton: Oliver Hazard Perry Throck Morton (1823-1877). He ran unsuccessfully in 1856 for governor of Indiana as a Republican but was elected lieutenant governor in 1860. When Governor Henry S. Lane was picked for the U.S. Senate, Morton became governor and was re-elected in 1864. He was a strong unionist and indefatigable wartime organizer known as a friend to soldiers. He was elected to fill out Henry Lane's unexpired term as a U.S. Senator and re-elected in 1873. He died in office in 1877.

Col. Thomas H. Bringhurst: Residence: Logansport, Indiana. Date of commission as major: 30 September 1861. Date of muster: 11 December 1861. Date of commission as lieutenant colonel: 25 May 1862; date of muster: 26 May 1862. Date of muster and date of commission as colonel: 6 August 1862. Mustered out with the regiment. Bringhurst succeeded Graham N. Fitch as commanding officer of the 46th Indiana in August 1862 after Fitch had to retire because of an incapacitating injury.

Dr. Jessup: Robert B. Jessup, Surgeon, Indiana 24th. Residence: Vincennes, Indiana. Date of muster: 31 July 1861. Date of commission: 13 August 1861. Resigned 25 September 1863.

Dr. Castlebury: Isaac Casselberry, Surgeon, First Cavalry, (28th Regiment) Indiana Volunteers. Residence: Evansville, Indiana. Date of commission: 13 August 1861. Date of muster: 20 August 1861.

Reese Laird: Reese D. Laird, Pvt., Co. B, Indiana 46th. Died at Memphis, Tennessee 13 December 1862, as a result of gunshot wounds.

Sunday Night Dec. 21st

Yesterday Col. Bringhurst went home on furlough. This morning a large number of transports arrived loaded with troops – been coming all day – 72 are said to be here and on the route. Two divisions of this army, Steele's and Washburn's Cavalry Division it is said will also accompany the expedition. This will swell the number of troops to at least sixty thousand. Vicksburg is thought to be the point of attack. Six Ohio Regts 14th, 16th, 42nd, 54th, 114th, and 120th I have seen to day. In the 120th Co. I - I found an old acquaintance Ad. Morrow from Richland County. Had a long chat with him. Had not seen him since the winter I formed his acquaintance in 1857-8. Gen. Sherman commands the expedition. Gen. Blair also accompanies it. Gen. Gorman is in command of this district. Having been rebrigaded we are now in the 1st Brig. 2nd Division instead of 2nd Brigade 4th Division as before. Brig. Gen. A.T. Hovey is still our division commander.

NOTES FOR December 21

Ad. Morrow: Alexander Morrow, 2nd Lt., Co. I, Ohio 120th; date of commission 13 August 1862. Resigned 18 February 1863. Underhill and Morrow probably attended Madison College together.

Gen. Sherman: (Union) General William Tecumseh Sherman (1820-1891).

Gen. Blair: (Union) Brigadier General Francis P. (Frank) Blair, Jr. (1821-1875), was the son of Francis P. Blair, Sr. (1791-1876), a Kentucky newspaperman who had moved to Washington to edit the *Washington Globe* and became an advisor of sorts to Lincoln. A graduate of Princeton and Transylvania Law School, Frank Blair was a lawyer in St. Louis who helped keep Missouri in the Union. He was a representative to Congress from Missouri but also held a commission in Sherman's army and was later promoted to major general. His brother Montgomery Blair (1813-1883) was Postmaster in Lincoln's cabinet until his resignation was requested on September 23, 1864.

Gen. Gorman: (Union) Brigadier General Willis A. Gorman (1816-1876) relieved Brigadier General Steele in command at

Helena. He was born in Kentucky and went on to become a member of the Indiana bar and a state legislator. He had fought in the Mexican War and for a time was a territorial governor of Minnesota. He had also served in Congress.[6]

Dec. 23

Before dark last night the last boat had left on its way down the river. Our division is the only one left here. Yesterday wrote a letter to my aunt Rachel Johnson a resident of Snow Hill, Worcester Co: Maryland. I never have seen her and have not heard from her directly for many years. To-day I wrote home, also wrote Jno. Dixon Burnetts' Creek, Indiana.

NOTES FOR December 23
Rachel (Underhill) Johnson (b. ca. 1810 d. 1887) was an older sister of Underhill's father. She married John C. Johnson September 1, 1831. She resided at Snow Hill, Worcester County, Maryland, and is buried there.

Burnett's Creek: the post office for Burnettsville, Indiana.

Outpost near Helena Ark's. Christmas Night

Yesterday afternoon we received unexpected orders to move immediately to the outposts. Accordingly we packed up and left instanter. We are now on the road leading to White River and about three miles from the Mississippi River. We are encamped by the side of the 34th Ind Col. Cameron. About ¾ mile from the pickets. We have pleasant camp on a gently rolling piece of ground, but water is scarce. The boys are in no gentle humor about leaving their comfortable quarters. Christmas been dull – engaged principally in finishing the move ordered yesterday. One year ago to-day was encamped on Beech Fork of Salt River, near Bardstown, Ky. Weather to day warm and rainy. Had a thunder storm.

NOTES FOR December 25
Col. Cameron: Robert Alexander Cameron, 34th Indiana. Residence: Valparaiso, Indiana. Date of commission and muster: 15 June 1862. Promoted to brigadier general, 11 August 1863. Before the war he was for a time a medical student, then published the *Valparaiso Republican.* He attended the 1860 Republican convention. He fought at New Madrid, Island No. 10, Vicksburg, Jackson, and during the Red River Campaign. He was brevetted major general of volunteers. Later he settled in Colorado.[7]

Outpost. Helena Ark.
Saturday Night Dec 27th

Heavy thunder storm to-day. Hail fell. Weather warm. Have our tent put up on left wing. Thought some of taking certain negro-quarters nearby for hospital, but after fitting them gave up the notion. Send our worst sick to Genrl. Hospital to-morrow. Balance of our sick back at our old camp ground under care of Dr. Washburn. Rumors are afloat that we will be soon removed from Helena. Pickets fired upon by guirrillas almost every night. None of our Regt lately hurt by them. No news yet from the fleet that a few days since went down the river. First news received to day of changes in the Cabinet. We suffer more through the quarrels and jealousies of leaders civil as well as military, than we do from defeats by our enemies. If our country yet goes to perdition it will be the fault of men in high civil and military trust and not of the people or army as a mass.

Rec'd yesterday number of Jeffersonian, and to-night wrote John Dixon.

NOTES FOR December 27
the Cabinet: Lincoln's cabinet was singularly inharmonious but represented different factions within the Republican party. It comprised William H. Seward, Secretary of State; Salmon P. Chase, Secretary of the Treasury; Edward Bates, Attorney General; Caleb B. Smith, Secretary of the Interior;

Montgomery Blair, Postmaster General; Gideon Welles, Secretary of the Navy; and Simon Cameron, Secretary of War. Charges of fraud and mismanagement swirled around Cameron, who failed to take Lincoln's hints to resign. In January 1862, after Cameron issued a statement about slavery without Lincoln's authorization, Lincoln fired him and replaced him with Edwin Stanton. Caleb B. Smith, who had been disaffected for some time with Lincoln's policies and suffering ill health as well, resigned in November 1862 to be replaced by Assistant Secretary of the Interior, John P. Usher.

Chase and Seward were bitter rivals. Welles had helped defeat Seward for the Republican presidential nomination and did not like Stanton. Blair was disliked by Thurlow Weed, a close ally of Seward's. Blair disliked Chase and and had complained to Lincoln about Stanton.

In December 1862, a cabinet crisis erupted. Chase had been quietly telling certain senators that cabinet meetings were disorganized, that members were not properly consulted before decisions were made, that Seward frequently failed to attend. On December 16, Seward and his son, Frederick, Assistant Secretary of State, came to Lincoln with their resignations after a stinging attack by Republican senators, whose information had come largely from Chase, Seward's bitter rival. On December 18 a committee representing the Senate caucus met with Lincoln at the White House to urge him to make changes in his cabinet which would ensure the loyalty to him of all its members. They departed feeling confident changes would be made and that Seward at last would be ousted. Lincoln then brought the cabinet and the committee to the White House and challenged the committee to ask the cabinet if their charges were true. Chace was on the spot: if he supported the committee, his disloyalty to Lincoln would be clear. If he supported Lincoln, he would lose credibility with the committee. In the end, the cabinet declared the charges untrue and supported Lincoln. Chase offered to resign, as did Stanton. Lincoln immediately refused Stanton's resignation and then refused Chase's as well as the earlier ones from Seward and his son. After that, Seward and Chase knew they served at Lincoln's pleasure and

Lincoln affirmed control of his cabinet.

Underhill may have read of the quarrels and charges and also of Cameron's and Smith's departures but may not have known then that Lincoln had retained his other cabinet members.

Monday night Dec. 29th

Yesterday and to-day the weather pleasant. To night it has commenced raining – weather warm. Wrote a letter to Linnie yesterday. Last night 35 of our pickets were gobbled up by the Secesh on the St. Francis road without the firing of a gun. Since we have moved out here our medical quiz has been broken up, probably not to be resumed.

NOTES FOR December 29

Linnie: See November 4 note for Lina.

St. Francis road: A period map shows an Upper St. Francis Road and Old St. Francis Road. Both ran northeast out of Helena. Underhill's reference is not clear enough to determine which one he meant.

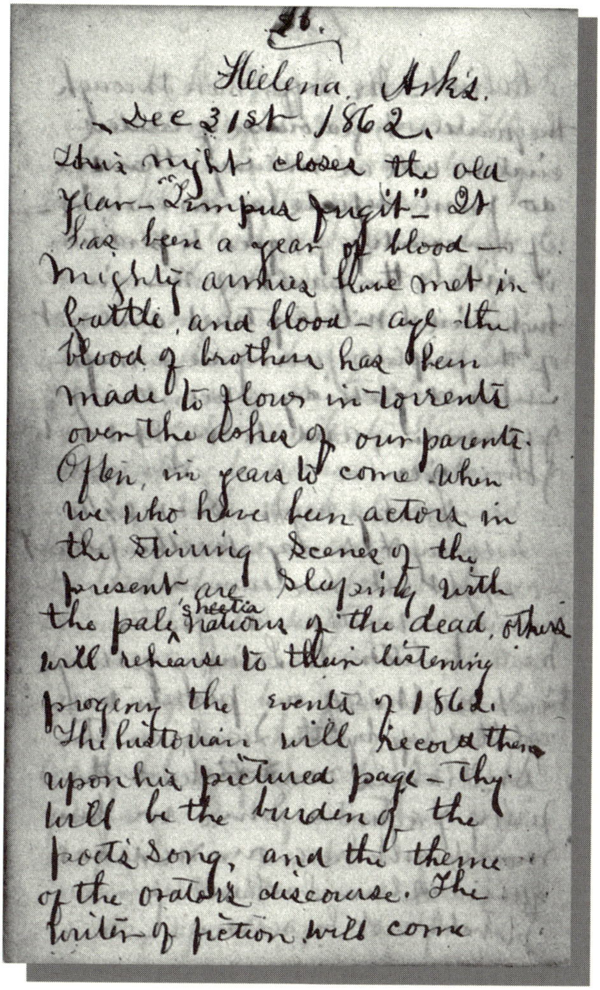
26.
Helena, Arks.
Dec 31st 1862.
This night closes the old
Year – "Tempus fugit" – It
has been a year of blood –
mighty armies have met in
battle, and blood – aye the
blood of brothers has been
made to flow in torrents
over the ashes of our parents.
Often, in years to come when
we who have been actors in
the stirring scenes of the
present are sleeping with
the pale sheetia nations of the dead, others
will rehearse to their listening
progeny the events of 1862.
The historian will record them
upon his pictured page – they
will be the burden of the
poets song, and the theme
of the orators discourse. The
writer of fiction will come

Helena, Arks.
Dec 31st 1862

This night closes the old year – "Tempus fugit –" It has been a year of blood. Mighty armies have met in battle, and blood – aye – the blood of brothers has been made to flow in torrents over the ashes of our parents. Often, in years to come when we who have been actors in the stirring scenes of the present are sleeping with the pale sheeted nations of the dead, others will rehearse to their listening progeny the events of 1862. The historian will record them upon his pictured page. They will be the burden of the poet's song, and the theme of the orator's discourse. The writer of fiction will come . . .

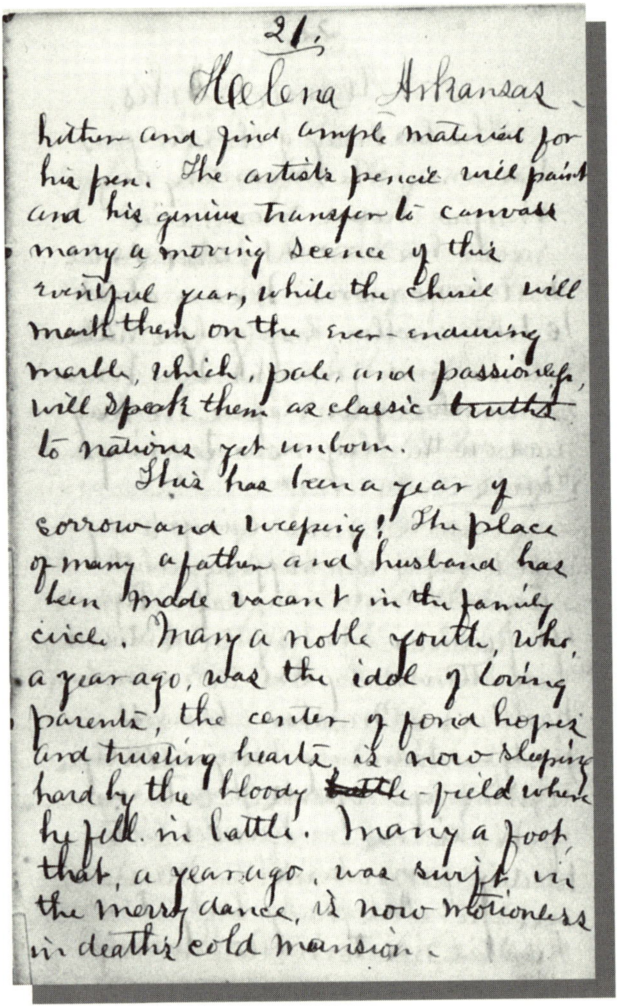

21,

Helena Arkansas.

hither and find ample material for his pen. The artists pencil will paint and his genius transfer to canvass many a moving scence of this eventful year, while the chisil will mark them on the ever-enduring marble, which, pale, and passionless, will speak them as classic ~~truths~~ to nations yet unborn.

This has been a year of sorrow and weeping! The place of many a father and husband has been made vacant in the family circle. Many a noble youth, who, a year ago, was the idol of loving parents, the center of fond hopes and trusting hearts, is now sleeping hard by the bloody ~~battle~~-field where he fell in battle. Many a foot, that, a year ago, was swift in the merry dance, is now motionless in deaths cold mansion.

. . . hither and find ample material for his pen. The artist's pencil will paint and his genius transfer to canvass many a moving scene of this eventful year, while the chisil will mark them on the ever-enduring marble, which, pale, and passionless, will speak them as classic truths to nations yet unborn.

This has been a year of sorrow and weeping! The place of many a father and husband has been made vacant in the family circle. Many a noble youth, who, a year ago, was the idol of loving parents, the center of fond hopes, and trusting hearts, is now sleeping hard by the bloody field where he fell in battle. Many a foot, that, a year ago, was swift in the merry dance, is now motionless in death's cold mansion. . . .

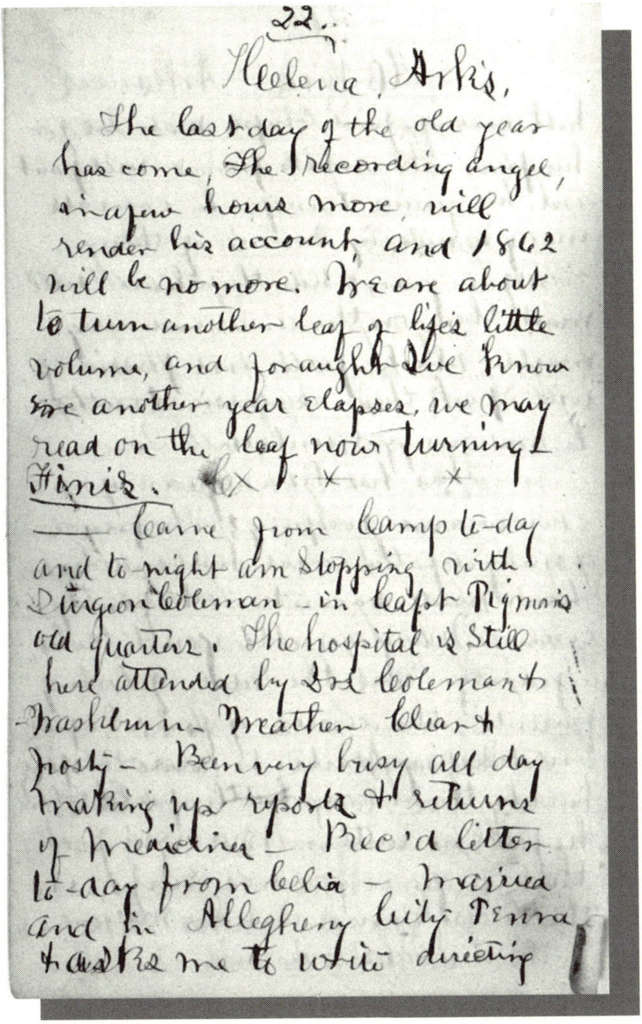
22.
Helena, Arks,
The last day of the old year has come, The recording angel, in a few hours more, will render his account, and 1862 will be no more. We are about to turn another leaf of life's little volume, and for aught I've known ere another year elapses, we may read on the leaf now turning Finis. x x x
Came from camp to-day and to-night am stopping with Surgeon Coleman in Capt Pigman's old quarters. The hospital is still here attended by Drs Coleman & Washburn. Weather clear & frosty – Been very busy all day making up reports & returns of medicines – Rec'd letter to-day from Celia – married and in Allegheny City Penna & asks me to write directing

The last day of the old year has come, the recording angel, in a few hours more, will render his account, and 1862 will be no more. We are about to turn another leaf of life's little volume, and for aught I've known ere another year elapses, we may read on the leaf now turning – Finis.

* * *

Came from camp to-day and to-night am stopping with Surgeon Coleman in Capt. Pigman's old quarters. The hospital is still here attended by Drs Coleman and Washburn. Weather clear and frosty. Been very busy all day making up reports and returns of medicines. Rec'd letter to-day from Celia – married and in Allegheny City, Tenna and asks me to write directing . . .

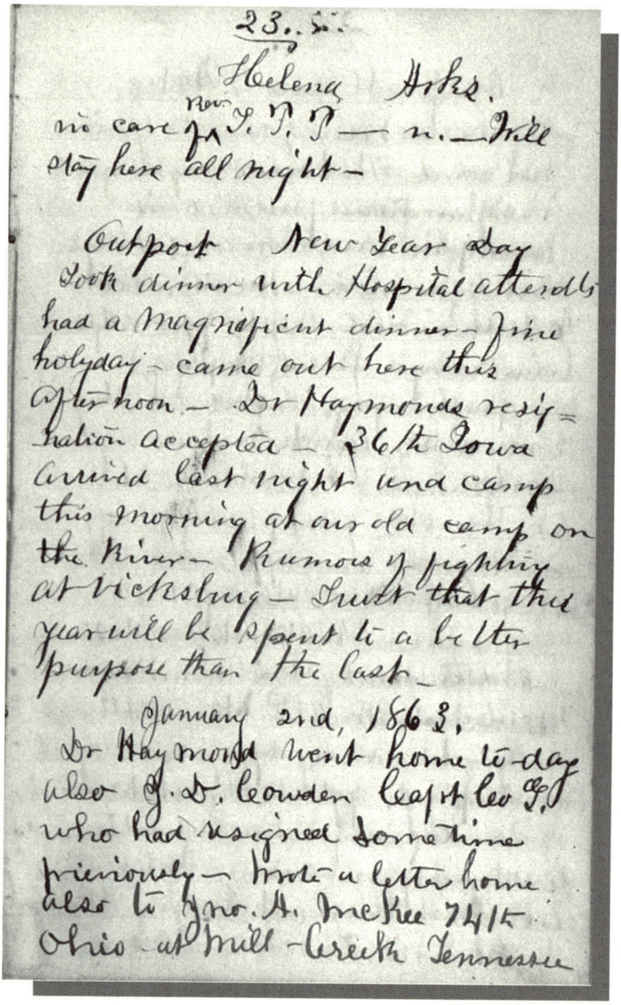
23..

Helena Arks.
in care of Rev. L. T. T— n.— Will
stay here all night—

Outpost New Year Day
Took dinner with Hospital attendts
had a magnificent dinner— fine
holyday— came out here this
afternoon— Dr Haymonds resig-
nation accepted— 36th Iowa
arrived last night and camp
this morning at our old camp on
the River— Rumors of fighting
at Vicksburg— Trust that this
year will be spent to a better
purpose than the last—

January 2nd, 1863.
Dr Haymond went home to-day
also J. D. Cowden Capt Co G.
who had resigned some time
previously— Wrote a letter home
also to Jno. A. McKee 74th
Ohio at Mill-Creek Tennessee

Helena, Arks.

. . . in care of Rev. L.T. T.___n. Will stay here all night—

Outpost New Year Day

Took dinner with hospital attendants. Had a magnificent dinner – fine holyday. Came out here this afternoon. Dr Haymonds resignation accepted. 36th Iowa arrived last night and camp this morning at our old camp on the river. Rumors of fighting at Vicksburg. Trust that this year will be spent to a better purpose than the last.

January 2nd, 1863.

Dr. Haymond went home to-day, also J. D. Cowdin, Capt. Co. G. who had resigned some time previously. Wrote a letter home, also to Jno. A. McKee 74th Ohio at Mill Creek Tennessee.

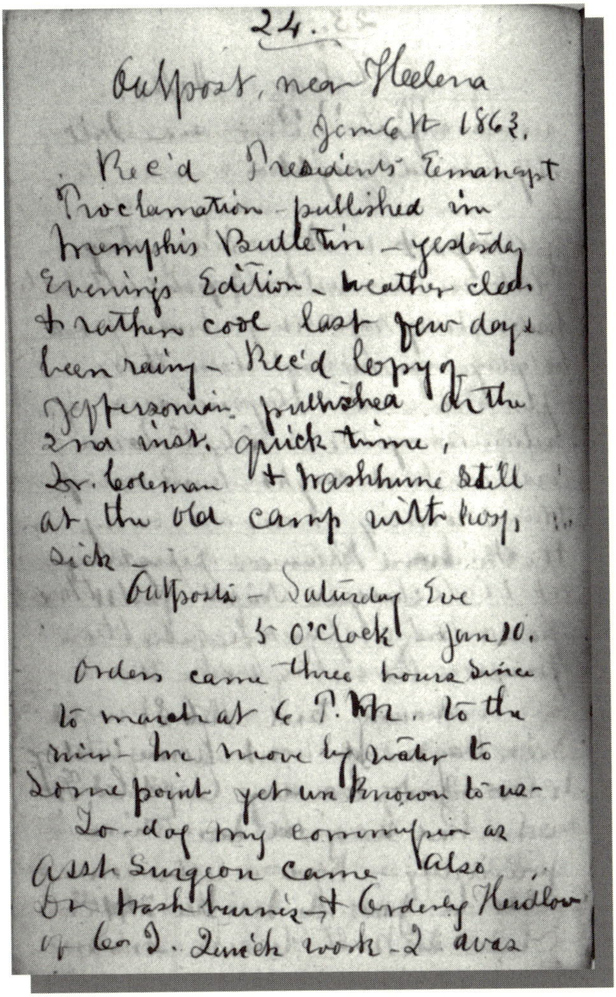
24.
Outpost, near Helena
Jan 6th 1863.
Rec'd President's Emancipt
Proclamation published in
Memphis Bulletin – yesterday
Evening's Edition – weather clear
& rather cool last few days
been rainy – Rec'd copy of
Jeffersonian published on the
2nd inst. quick time,
Dr. Coleman & Washburne still
at the old camp with hosp,
sick
Outposts – Saturday Eve
5 O'clock Jan 10.
Orders came three hours since
to march at 6 P.M. to the
river – we move by water to
some point yet unknown to us –
To-day my commission as
Asst Surgeon came also
Dr Washburne's & Orderly Hudlow
of Co. I. Quick work – I was

Outpost, near
Helena
Jan 6th 1863

Rec'd President's Emancipt. Proclamation published in Memphis Bulletin – yesterday evening's edition. Weather clear and rather cool – last few days been rainy. Rec'd copy of Jeffersonian published on the 2nd inst. Quick time. Dr. Coleman and Washburne still at the old camp with hosp. sick.

Outposts – Saturday Eve
5 o'clock Jan. 10

Orders came three hours since to march at 6 P.M. to the river. We move by water to some point yet unknown to us. To-day my commission as Asst Surgeon came, also Dr. Washburne's and Orderly Hudlow of Co. I. Quick work – I was . . .

. . . not expecting a return so soon. All our medical stores and everything of the kind has been removed to the river. I am sitting in the open air and writing on my knee. Weather warm and pleasant. No news from Vicksburg, but rumors of a bloody victory achieved by Gen. Rosecrans in Tennessee near Murfreesboro. Nothing definite. Perhaps in another hour we will be at the river.

NOTES FOR December 31

Capt. Pigman: William A. Pigman. Residence: Delphi, Indiana. Commissioned first lieutenant 4 October 1861. Date of commission and muster as captain: 1 July 1862. Wounded at Sabine Cross Roads. Honorably discharged 18 December 1864.

Rev. L.T. T___n.: The initials of the Reverend are not easy to read and are educated guesses.

NOTES FOR January 2

John A. McKee was a college friend. He probably attended Madison College with Underhill but Muskingum College has a record of a John A. McKee from Cambridge enrolled in the Scientific Department of the Muskingum College Preparatory Department in 1857-8. A second lieutenant in the Ohio 74th, Company K, he drowned in Cincinnati February 1, 1864.

NOTES FOR January 6

Emancipt. Proclamation: The Emancipation Proclamation. In September 1862, Lincoln had issued a preliminary proclamation stating that emancipation would take place on January 1, 1863. The Emancipation Proclamation freed slaves in states fighting against the Union, not slaves in border states on the Union side nor in southern areas controlled by the Union. Only the 13th Amendment to the Constitution enacted in December 1865 ended slavery for all in the United States.

inst.: of the present month.

NOTES FOR January 10

Orderly Hudlow, Co. I.: Jacob Hudlow, Sergeant. Enlisted 2 December 1861. Commissioned second lieutenant 30 December

1862. Killed at Sabine Cross Roads, Louisiana, 8 April 1864. No posthumous promotion.

Gen. Rosecrans: (Union) Major General William Starke Rosecrans (1819-1898) graduated from West Point in 1842, staying in the Army until 1854, when he went into business. He came back to the Army in 1861. After the war he was a minister to Mexico from 1867-69 and a congressman from California from 1881-1885.

Murfreesboro: A town in Tennessee two miles southeast of the scene of fierce fighting at Stones River from 31 December 1862 until 3 January 1863. Forces under General William S. Rosecrans, who had assumed command of the Army of the Cumberland from Don Carlos Buell, were attacked by Confederate forces under Major General Bragg. After heavy fighting and steep losses on both sides, the Confederates retreated on January 3 twenty-five miles south, giving the Union a much-needed victory and a boost to morale. This action was almost simultaneous with Sherman's abortive assault at Chickasaw Bayou, launched December 29.

on board Steamer "Sunshine"
Sabbath Night Jan 11-1863

Last night we marched on board. Did not get our stores all on board till late at night. Sick last night and been confined to bed nearly all day. Better to-night however. Left Helena this evening a little after sunset. A sufficient garrison will be left to hold the fort and town. Only a portion of the steamers left with us. Balance will probably soon follow. My commission was handed me this morning by the Adjutant. It reads "appointed Vice Ast. Surgeon. Haymond resigned" and dated Dec. 30. Dr. Washburne's – "Vice Ast. Surgeon Spencer resigned" dated Dec. 26. To-day I am twenty six years old! Time flies, alas, how swiftly! A little while ago and I was a careless happy child playing among the flowers and pleasant fields of my dear old home! How well do I remember the winding creek along whose green banks I have spent many joyous hours angling for minnows, the grand old forest with its gnarled oaks spreading beeches and beautiful maples, the deep mossy spring, and every loved object my infancy knew. But those days are gone never to return. This recollection will remain green on the tablet of memory forever.

NOTES FOR January 11
Sunshine: a side-wheel packet built at Elizabeth, Pennsylvania in 1860. She was torched at St. Louis in July 1864.[8]

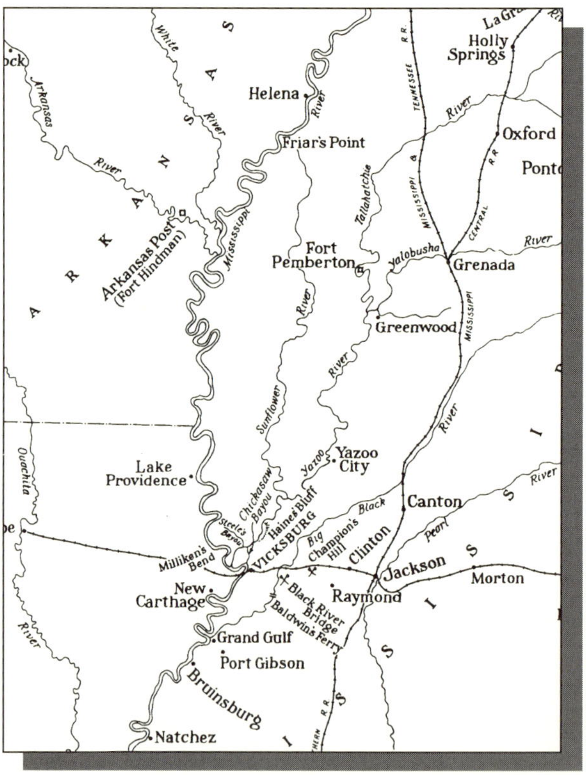

Mississippi Shore – Opposite mouth of White River Monday morning – Jan 12. 1863–

Arrived here last night and lay up to shore. All the steamers some 15 in number are now here. We will now proceed up White River – at least as far as the cut off. This is the fourth trip for our Reg't up that river. On the 16 of July last we came out of White River and proceeded up to Helena. One year ago to-day we were in Camp Wickliff Ky and I was on detached duty as surgeon of 15th Ind. Infantry. Yesterday I wrote a note home before leaving Helena. Weather exceedingly fine and pleasant.

NOTES FOR January 12
Camp Wickliffe: Named after former governor Charles Wickliffe, this was an assembly camp for Union regiments in LaRue County, Kentucky, about five miles east of Hodgenville, a little north of Buffalo, along McDougall's Creek, in existence only from December 1861 until February 1862.

White River Prairie Landing
Tuesday morn. Jan 13.

Arrived here yesterday eve and lay all night. 23 miles from the Mississippi and 60 from St. Charles. Instead of 15 we have about 30 transports. Gen. Gorman came up last night. Brings reports of the capture of Arkansas Post. We proceed up the river this morning. Some cavalry have landed and go up on western side of the river. A large body of cavalry go across from Helena to the river at some point above. Had an interesting game of poker last night.

NOTES FOR January 13
St. Charles: A small town of about two hundred located in northeast Arkansas on the White River, according to Underhill about eighty-four miles from its mouth. An historical marker close to the river notes where the shot was fired that hit the USS *Mound City*, a shot considered one of the most destructive of the war. A monument in the center of the main street commemorates both Union and Confederate soldiers.

Steamer "Sunshine"–
off St. Charles, White River
Jan. 14

Last night we lay off Indian Bay and put out pickets on the western side of the river. Reconnoitering revealed that the enemy has evacuated the place. This morning we have stopped here. On the 17th of last June our regiment had a brilliant little fight here at the same time the terrible disaster occurred to the gun boat Mound City. Heavy rain last night. Still raining heavily this morning.

January 14
Mound City: The *Mound City* was one of seven Union city-class gunboats belonging to the Mississippi Squadron and was built at Mound City, Illinois. The city-class gunboats were named after western river ports. (See note for *Cincinnati*, January 16.) On 17 June 1862, before Underhill's diary opens, three gunboats, *St. Louis*, *Lexington*, and *Conestoga*, and a transport with Underhill's regiment aboard, under the command of Colonel Fitch, had gone on an expedition up the White River in Arkansas to open communications with General Curtis. The gunboats were fired upon and the *Mound City* took a hit in the main steam line. Only 23 of the 175 men aboard escaped scalding. Many jumped overboard and were shot in the water or drowned. At the back of the diary is a poem which commemorates this.

Off St. Charles – Jan. 15, 1863

Well, we are still lying here where we lay the greater portion of yesterday. However we will move on up the river in the course of an hour. Rained all day yesterday and part of last night. Toward morning got colder and commenced snowing. Still snowing a little this morning. Snow more than an inch deep. Second and heaviest snow we have had this season. Weather pretty cold – – Yesterday several buildings were burned in St. Charles. Heavy breastworks had been thrown up around a portion of the town by the Rebel force. Breastworks surrounded by deep ditch. Several heavy guns had been mounted but all were moved to Post Arkansas before the fight there. Considerable sickness is occurring in the regiment as a consequence of crowding so many men together. Quite sick myself last night but on duty this morning.

Steamer "Sunshine"
January 16. Afternoon

Cold and clear to-day. Snow four inches deep. We are now 15 miles above Clarendon or 150 from the Mississippi. Our cavalry day before yesterday reached Clarendon from Helena, had a skirmish with a few cavalry and captured a number of them. The Steamer "Blue Wing" captured by the Secesh about the time of the late Vicksburg expedition is only a few hours ahead of us. Rocket has been despatched after her but will probably not overtake her. The river is high and in excellent boating condition. Very crooked. We make some turns where we can see boats only a few hundred yards distant from us by land, but perhaps more than five miles distant by water. The country is not so low and marshy as below. Bluffs are frequently seen. Duvall's is most likely our immediate destination. Gen. Benton is reported at Jacksonport. Also Gen. Blunt reported 15 miles from Little Rock and supplies cut off. Card playing has been principal amusement till yesterday when it was broken up by an order from Lieut. Col. Gould Commanding Regt. No smoking allowed on boat by order of Gen. Gorman Commander of expedition. Yesterday two gunboats – Cincinnati and Baron de Kalb overtook us at St. Charles. Yesterday completed a thorough review of "Sargent's Minor Surgery."

NOTES FOR January 16
Clarendon: a town in Arkansas and the seat of Monroe County, on the White River roughly 135 miles from the mouth of the Mississippi and about fifty miles upstream from St. Charles.

Blue Wing: a side-wheel packet built at Jeffersonville, Indiana in 1850. A U.S. gunboat seized her December 10, 1862 when those aboard were charged with trading with the enemy. She was taken to Helena, Arkansas and placed in the U.S. Quartermaster Department. About December 20, 1862, she left Memphis for the Yazoo and en route, was hijacked by the Confederates on the Mississippi River at Napoleon and taken up the Arkansas River to Arkansas Post. Federal troops later recaptured much of the ammunition aboard. *Way's Packet Directory, 1848-1994*, alleges she was burned at Arkansas Post December 28,

1862, but Underhill's entry shows that this is incorrect.[9]

Rocket : a stern-wheel packet built at Brownsville, Pennsylvania in 1856 that was in government service most of the war.[10]

Duvall's Bluff: a small Arkansas town on the White River, according to Underhill 176 miles from its mouth.

Gen. Benton: (Union) Brigadier General William Plummer Benton (1828-1867) was born in Maryland and had fought in the Mexican War. At the time of this entry he was commanding the 1st Division, Army of Southeast Missouri, department of the Missouri. He had fought at Pea Ridge, Arkansas, and later was slightly wounded at Jackson, Mississippi. He died of yellow fever in New Orleans.[11]

Jacksonport: in Jackson County, Arkansas, on the White River, 357 miles from its mouth, according to Underhill, and about twenty-five miles southeast of Batesville.

Gen. Blunt: (Union) Major General James G. Blunt (1826-1881) was born in Maine, graduated from the Starling Medical College, and moved in 1856 to Kansas, where he became an active abolitionist. He worked with John Brown getting slaves into Canada.

Lt. Col. Gould: John H. Gould. Residence: Delphi, Indiana. Date of commission as captain: 4 October 1861. Date of muster: 1 November 1861. Promoted to major. Date of commission and muster: 25 May 1862. Promoted to lieutenant colonel. Date of commission and muster: 6 August 1862. Resigned 9 February 1863. Re-entered the service as Lt. Col. 135th Regiment.

Cincinnati: One of seven city-class ironclad gunboats of the Mississippi Squadron ordered by the Army and constructed by James B. Eads (1820-1887). The *Cincinnati* was built in 45 days. Commissioned in January 1862, the city-class gunnboats were the first ironclads in the western hemisphere. They were 175 feet long, had a 51 foot beam, and drew 6 feet. They had 2.5 inch thick iron plating over laminated 12.5 to 24 inch oak. The center paddle wheel was concealed. They were designed to fight bow on. The others were: *Pittsburg, Louisville; St. Louis,* later renamed the *Baron De Kalb*; *Carondelet,* after Carondelet, Missouri, a small town on the Mississippi about ten miles south of St. Louis which was annexed by the city in 1870; *Mound City,* after Mound City, Illinois, a town about seven miles upstream on the Ohio River from Cairo; and *Cairo*, named after Cairo, Illinois, located at the junction of the Ohio and Mississippi Rivers, the town watched for in the night by Mark Twain's Huck and Jim, so they could take a steamboat into free territory. The *Cairo* was sunk in the Yazoo River by Confederates using the newly-developed torpedo 12 December 1862. The vessel was found in 1964 and raised off the bottom. What remains of it can be seen today in the Vicksburg Military Park.

Baron De Kalb: a city-class gunboat of the Mississippi squadron, formerly the USS *St. Louis*, built at St. Louis.

Sargent's Minor Surgery: most likely *Principles and Practice of Modern Surgery* (1848), edited by Fitz William Sargent, also known as *Druitt's Modern Surgery* by Robert Druitt. Interestingly, Sargent was the father of artist John Singer Sargent.

Duvall's Bluff
Saturday morning Jan 17

Arrived here yesterday evening. Secesh left after our boats hove in sight. Went towards Little Rock. Captured about a dozen prisoners, three large guns and a quantity of small arms – pretty well fortified – Weather cold this morning but moderating some.

Jan 18

Still lying here, probably go down the river to-morrow. Weather moderating – snow partly melted away. Religious service this (Sabbath) morning conducted in the back cabin by our Chaplain, the Rev. Hamilton Robb. Dispatches rec'd from Helena to day. Squad bringing dispatches attacked by guirrellas. 7 killed and 15 captured. Messenger arrived safe at Clarendon and was then brought up by the steamer Anderson on her way from St. Charles where several boats had been left. Character of dispatches said to be that we must rendezvous at Napoleon where an immense army will be massed to move against Vicksburg. Wrote a note home yesterday – first opportunity of mailing letter since we left Helena.

NOTES FOR January 18
Anderson: most likely the *General Anderson*, a side-wheel packet built at Brownsville, Pennsylvania in 1860. Originally on the Nashville-Cairo run, the Union seized it early in the war.[12]

Napoleon: a town on the west bank of the Mississippi in Arkansas where the Arkansas River empties into the Mississippi. Today the town no longer exists but at the time of the Civil War, it had several thousand inhabitants and a large military hospital.

St. Charles – Tuesday morning January 20

Yesterday morning left the Bluff and lay a few miles above this place last night. At Clarendon met the mail boat – first mail rec'd for the trip. Rec'd letter from Linnie and paper from White County. Last night was up till late with a sick man – Theodore Stringham private Co: K – died in two or three hours from time he took sick. Atmosphere is a little chilly this morning. Weather cloudy.

NOTES FOR January 20
White County: the county in Indiana where Underhill was living when he enlisted.

Theodore W. Stringham, Pvt., Co. K. Residence: Green Oak, Indiana. Date of muster: 11 December 1861. Died at St. Charles, Arkansas, 20 January 1863.

Steamer "Sunshine"
Mississippi River Jan. 21st

Passed out of White River about noon and are now on our way up to Helena again. Much disappointed that we did not get the opportunity of going on down to Vicksburg. Met a portion of Grant's army on their way down. Snow entirely gone and weather mild and spring like. Been reading to-day "Count Robert of Paris" one of the "Waverly Novels" by Walter Scott. Like all the rest of his novels it is a very entertaining book.

NOTES FOR January 21
Grant: (Union) General Ulysses S. Grant (1822-1885).

In Camp near Helena Ark's.
Jan. 25, 1863

Arrived at Helena 22nd. Lay on the Mississippi shore opposite Helena all night. Next morning moved to this side and camped on river bank. In the afternoon were ordered back of town and came out here yesterday. Are now camped on the steep hill sides just back of town. Very muddy been raining several days and still very disagreeable. Last mail received letter from George Spencer – also note from Sallie H. of Richland Co. Result of expedition may thus be summed up: Cost about one million, a great deal wear and tear and accomplished the unnecessary feat of burning a number of out-houses at various places along the river. This afternoon wrote two letters, one home and one to Linnie. Dr. Coleman to-day appointed Med. Director of 2nd division.

NOTES FOR January 25
Sallie H.: There is no information who she was. She might have been a college friend at Madison College. Mansfield is the county seat of Richland County, Ohio.

In Camp near Helena – Jan. 27

Yesterday completed "Count Robert of Paris." Like it well, but not so good as some others of Scotts.

—Principal Characters —

Alexsis Comnenus	*Emperor*
Irene	*Empress*
Anna Comnena	*Princess*
Caesar Nicephorus Briennius	*Prince*
Agelastes	*Courtier*
Achilles Tatius	*Capt. of Varangians*
Hereward	*The Faithful Varangian*
Count Robert	*The Crusader*
Brenhinda	*Countess*

To-day commenced reading "Castle Dangerous" by same author. Weather been rainy a week or so. Consequently roads and camp extremely muddy. Caught cold and rather unwell. Yesterday wrote Lieut. G.W. Spencer. Rec'd letter from home, also one from Aunt Rachel Johnson of Snow Hill, Worcester County, Maryland.

In Camp near Helena Ark's.
February 4, 1863

Since last paragraph was written have had fine weather clear and cold. To-day, however, it is snowing – third snow that has fell this winter. Frank Herman arrived yesterday. Made up Monthly Report for January on the 1st inst. and forwarded to Medical Director of Brigade. Been busy in our Department for last week. Private Clinton J. Armstrong died on the morning of the 2nd. To-day wrote a letter to Cousin George T. Wilson, Burnettsville Somerset Co: Maryland.

NOTES FOR February 4

Frank Herman: The Hermans lived in Burnettsville, Indiana. The 1860 census shows Franklin Herman, 55, a farmer born in Kentucky, and his wife, Mary A., 52, housekeeper, born in Pennsylvania. Three daughters lived in the same household: Mary, 21; Margaret 16; and Harriet, 14. Herman had settled in Burnettsvile in 1839 and had laid out the town of Burnettsville in 1854. Underhill probably is referring to Franklin Herman, 33, a merchant born in Ohio, who is listed in another household from what must be his father, living with his wife, Isabel, 33, also born in Ohio, and daughter Amanda, 7. Also in the household was Joseph, 18, a clerk, presumably his brother. Joseph was a corporal in Company F of the 46th who had been discharged February 2 because he had developed what was probably pulmonary tuberculosis. Frank may have come to help his brother home.

George T. Wilson (1819-1889): Underhill's first cousin and the son of Underhill's mother's sister, Betsy. Wilson was the eldest of seven, a farmer and a waterman (one who earns a living by fishing, crabbing, or oystering). In 1857 he bought out his siblings' shares in the 200 acre Wilson homestead in Burnettsville, Maryland for $600. In 1860 he married Emma Louisa Garrison (1841-1919). They had no children. They are buried in St. Paul's Cemetery in Marion, Maryland, which is very close to Burnettsville.

Feb'y 5, 1863.

Snow 2 inches deep but weather pleasant. Rec'd copy of "Jeffersonian" containing several letters from Murfreesboro fight. My time kept busily occupied. Health of Reg't tolerably good.

In Camp near Helena Arks.
Feb'y 7, 1863

To-day returns north Frank Herman send two letters by him one to Dr. Fleming and one to Jno. Dixon. Yesterday discharge papers were rec'd for the following men

John Cornis,	*Co A*	*disease*	*Albuminuria*
Thos. S. Long	*" H.*		*Diabetes*
David Haller	*" K.*		*Atrophy left leg*
Joseph A. Herman	*" F.*		*Incipient Phthisis*

NOTES FOR February 7

Dr. Fleming: The Cincinnati College of Medicine and Surgery roster shows both Underhill and a William Fleming, residence Ohio, as having graduated in 1861. While several other Flemings are listed among Civil War surgeons, none seems plausible. It may be that both Underhill and Fleming went to White County to practice, because the diary entries would suggest that Fleming had remained in Monticello or nearby and was not in the service. An AMA listing of deceased physicians lists him as an 1861 graduate of the Cincinnati College of Medicine and Surgery, an allopath, or general practitioner, and assumes a date of death of 31 December 1929.

John Cornis, Pvt., Co. A. Residence: Pittsburgh, Indiana. Date of muster: 1 November 1861. Discharged 5 February 1863 because of disability.

Thomas S. Long, Pvt., Co. H. Residence: South Bend, Indiana. Date of muster: 5 November 1861. Discharged 5 February 1863 because of disability.

David Haller, Recruit, Co. K. Residence: Kendalville. Date of muster: 28 October 1862. Discharged 5 February 1863 because of disability.

Joseph A. Herman, Cpl., Co. F. Residence: Burnettsville, Indiana. Date of muster: 14 November 1861. Discharged 2 February 1863 because of disability. See the entry for February 4.

phthisis: Several definitions are given in the medical dictionary but the most likely is pulmonary tuberculosis.

Feby 8, 1863

Finished "Castle Dangerous"
Principal Characters –
Lady Augusta de Berkly – Sir John de Walton – Aymer de Valence – Lady Margaret de Hautlieu – Malcolm Fleming – Sir James of Douglas. Also read "My Aunt Margaret's Mirror," "Tapestried Chamber" and "Death of Laird's Jock" all by the same author.

NOTES FOR February 8
Lady Augusta de Berkly. This should be the Lady Augusta Berkeley. "My Aunt Margaret's Mirror," "The Tapestried Chamber," and "The Laird's Jock" are short stories by Sir Walter Scott.

In camp, Near Helena, Ark's.
Feby 9.

Rec'd letter from Linnie dated January 17. Daniel Samsel Private - Co. D. discharged yesterday on account of gunshot wound. Weather mild.

NOTES FOR February 9
Daniel Samsel: See diary entry and note for October 27.

Feby 12.

Yesterday wrote home. G. W. Clinger – John A Nicholson, and Peter O'Farrell discharged 11th inst. Col. Gould's resignation accepted. Dr. Coleman gets leave of absence. Weather pleasant.

NOTES FOR February 12
G.W. Clinger, Pvt., Co. E. Residence: Royal Center, Indiana. Date of muster: 5 November 1861. Discharged 11 February 1863 because of disability.

John A. Nicholson, Pvt., Co. G. Residence: White City, Indiana. Date of muster: 5 November 1861. Discharged 11 February 1863 because of disability.

Peter O'Farrell, Pvt., Co. A. Residence: Prince William, Indiana. Date of muster: 11 November 1861. Discharged 11 February 1863 because of disability.

Feby 14.

This morning died Josiah Metz of Co. E. of pneumonia – ruined last night. To day one year ago Regt. left camp Wickliff Kentucky. Order rec'd this evening to leave to-morrow with 3 days rations – move supposed to be temporary.

NOTES FOR February 14

Josiah Metz, Pvt., Co. E. Residence: Burnettsville, Indiana. Date of muster: 15 November 1861. Metz would have been 18 or 19. In the 1860 census he is shown as age 16, a farm laborer, living with John Billings, 24, a farmer, and his wife Matilda, 18, and daughter Elizabeth, 1.

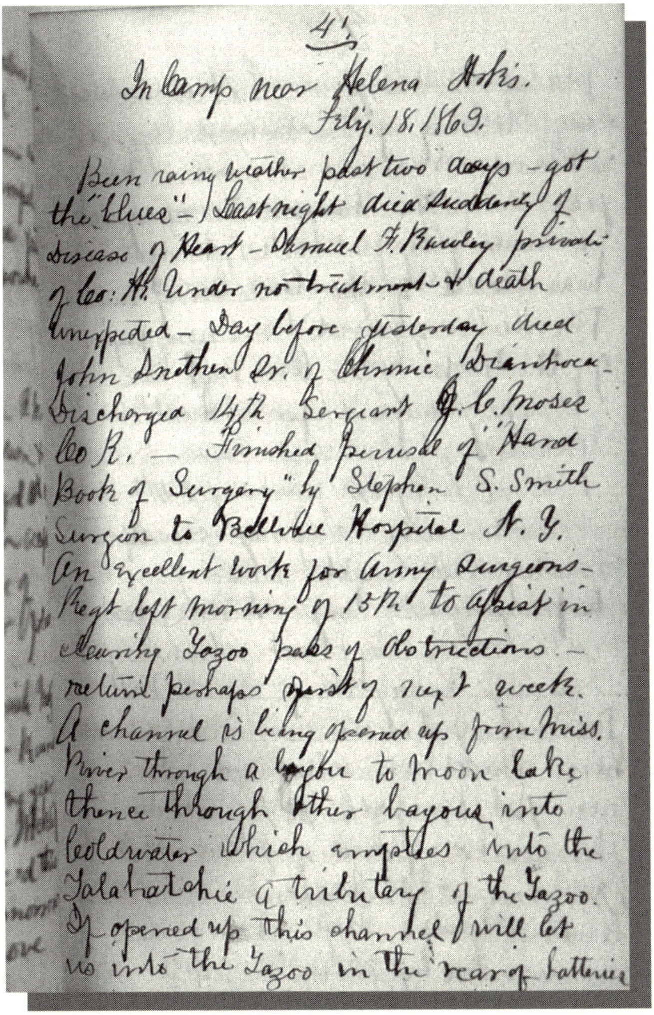

4

In Camp near Helena Ark's.
Feb'y. 18, 1863.

Been rainy weather past two days - got the "blues" - Last night died suddenly of disease of Heart - Samuel F. Rawley private of Co: H. Under no treatment & death unexpected - Day before yesterday died John Snethen Jr. of Chronic Diarrhoea - Discharged 14th Sergeant J. C. Moses Co K. - Finished perusal of "Hand Book of Surgery" by Stephen S. Smith Surgeon to Bellvue Hospital N. Y. An excellent work for Army Surgeons - Reg't left morning of 15th to assist in clearing Yazoo pass of obstructions - return perhaps first of next week. A channel is being opened up from Miss. River through a bayou to Moon lake thence through other bayous into Coldwater which empties into the Talahatchie a tributary of the Yazoo. If opened up this channel will let us into the Yazoo in the rear of batteries

In Camp near
Helena Ark's.
Feb'y 18, 1863.

Been rainy weather past two days – got the "blues–" Last night died suddenly of disease of the heart Samuel F. Rawley private of Co:H. Under no treatment and death unexpected. Day before yesterday died John Snethen Jr. of Chronic Diarrhoea. Discharged 14th Sergeant J. C. Moses Co.K. Finished perusal of "Hand Book of Surgery" by Stephen S. Smith Surgeon to Bellvue Hospital N.Y. An excellent work for Army surgeons. Reg't left morning of 15th to assist in clearing Yazoo pass of obstructions – return perhaps first of next week. A channel is being opened up from Miss. River through a bayou to Moon Lake, thence through other bayous, into Coldwater which empties into the Talahatchie a tributary of the Yazoo. If opened up this channel will let us into the Yazoo in the rear of batteries . . .

. . . placed on that river. The Rebels are busy blocking up the channel beyond where our men are at work. Many years since the channel was navigated particularly by flat boats. Navigation was closed by the levee being built. Paymasters arrived and are now paying off the troops here. Our Regt has not been paid for almost 6 months.

NOTES FOR February 18
Samuel F. Rawley, Recruit, Co. H. Died of heart disease at Helena, 17 February 1863.

John Snethen, Pvt., Co. C. Appointed wagoner. Died at Helena, Arkansas 16 February 1863.

J. C. Moses, Sgt., Co. K. Residence: Peru, Indiana. Date of muster: 12 November 1861. Discharged 14 February 1863 because of disability.

"Hand Book of Surgery" by Stephen S. Smith Surgeon to Bellvue Hospital N.Y.: Smith was born in 1823 in New York state and after studying in Buffalo, went to New York in 1849, where he studied at the College of Physicians and Surgeons, earning his MD in 1850. The book Underhill refers to was published in 1861-62 as a handbook of operations for surgeons in the field. It went through five printings. Smith held the chair of surgery at Bellevue Hospital and later became a professor of orthopedic surgery at the University of the City of New York. When Underhill attended Bellevue Hospital Medical College in 1865-66, Smith was on the faculty.

Yazoo pass: A waterway between Moon Lake and the Coldwater River. Because he could not take Vicksburg from the Mississippi River side because of many guns on its bluffs, General Grant was seeking a water route to get into the rear of Vicksburg. He cut a levee built some years before on the east side of the Mississippi opposite Helena, hoping to flood an area sufficiently to allow boats to reach the Yazoo river through Moon Lake, various bayous and lesser rivers. Many of these were overgrown and had to be cleared to allow boats to pass.

Moon Lake: A lake in Mississippi a short distance inland from the Mississippi River and only several miles east of Helena, Arkansas.

Coldwater: A river flowing south in northwestern Mississippi which joins the Little Tallahatchie to form the Tallahatchie River.

Talahatchie: The Tallahatchie River, which flows south in western Mississippi and joins with the Yallabusha River to form the Yazoo.

Yazoo: A major tributary flowing southwest through a cotton growing area of Mississippi and at the time of the Civil War, issuing into the Mississippi River about seven miles above Vicksburg. Bluffs along the Yazoo had been heavily fortified by the Confederates.

Feb'y 19

Weather dry and windy – ceased raining last night. Orders rec'd to prepare 15 days rations for another move. Regt not returned yet. Few days since Brig. Gen. B. M. Prentiss arrived and assumed command here. Have been rebrigaded. We are now 1st Brigade 13th Division. Brigade composed of 43rd, 46th and 47th Ind. 28th Wisconsin and 1st U.S. Regular Inf.– Brigade commanded by Brig. Gen. Solomon brother of Governor of Wisconsin. 2 brigades constitute the 13th Division commanded by Gen. Ross. Surg. George Hammond Medical Director of the District. Dr. Horace Coleman Medical Director of our division.

NOTES FOR February 19

Gen. B. M. Prentiss: (Union) Major General Benjamin M. Prentiss (1819-1901). Originally from Illinois, he had served in the Mexican War. He relieved Brigadier General Frederick Steele as post commander at Fort Curtis.

Brig. Gen. Soloman: (Union) Brigadier General Friedrich (Frederick) Sigel Salomon (1826-1897) built the fortifications at Fort Curtis. Frederick and his three brothers, Eberhardt, Edward, and Herman, were born in Saxony, leaving after 1848. Frederick, Eberhardt, and Edward had received military training in Germany. Frederick was trained as a surveyor and railroad engineer and Eberhardt as a civil engineer. Frederick eventually was brevetted a Union major general and Eberhardt was brevetted a Union brigadier general. Edward P. Salomon (1828-1909) was elected lieutenant governor of Wisconsin at age 33 and became Wisconsin's youngest governor when Governor Harvey died in 1862. Herman, the youngest brother, had not received military training in Germany but enlisted as a private on the Union side, re-enlisting after his three-year term expired. Their cousin, Edward Selig Saloman (1836-1913), was Colonel of the the Illinois 82nd, which fought at Gettysburg. He was brevetted a brigadier general.

Gen. Ross: (Union) Brigadier General Leonard Fulton Ross (1823-1901). An Illinois native and former Democratic politician, he had served in the Mexican War and left a law practice at the outbreak of the Civil War to become a regimental commander in the Union army. He became a brigadier general in April 1862. He resigned in July 1863, thinking the war nearly over.[13]

George Hammond – district medical director: George Hammond does not appear in any listing of Civil War Army doctors. Possibly John W. Hammond, who was Surgeon to the 120th Ohio Infantry. Like the Indiana 46th, the 120th Ohio was part of the Thirteenth Army Corps but in the Ninth, not the Twelfth Division. The 120th was at Young's Point, Louisiana between 17 January and 8 March, but Hammond may have remained behind at Helena.

Feby 25th, 1863.

Heavy thunder storm this morning. Regt paid off night before last. Yesterday our entire division left down the Yazoo Pass. Perhaps be gone two or three weeks. Regt only returned day before leaving one man – Private George Bruington Co. B. – was wounded in Coldwater – wound received in calf of left leg. Isaac Castle and John Stradley discharged a few days ago.

NOTES FOR February 25

George W. Bruington, Pvt., Co. B. Residence: Logansport, Indiana. Promoted to corporal. Wounded by guerrillas at the mouth of Yazoo Pass, 22 February 1863. Date of muster: 5 November 1861. Veteran mustered out 4 September 1865.

Isaac K. Castle, Sgt., Company B. Residence: Logansport, Indiana. Date of muster: 5 November 1861. Discharged 22 February 1863 because of disability.

John Stradley, Musician, Pvt., Company K. Residence: Rochester, Indiana. Date of muster: 11 December 1861. Discharged 20 February 1863 because of disability.

March 1.

To-day attended Divine service in Fort Curtis – short sermons were made by Rev. J. G. Forman Post Chaplain, Rev Sawyer, Chaplain 47th, and also by Chaplain of 28th Wisconsin. Proff. Hibbin, Chaplain of 11th Ind made a stirring patriotic address. The Proff. is a young man= slight form – pleasing address – with a romantic look remembering me of the pictures of Byron. A graduate of some Indiana institution and for a short time filled a chair in a Literary College. He is a minister of the Methodist Denomination. Weather, warm and pleasant – roads drying up – Spring has fairly set in. Wrote a letter home few days since. To-morrow must write Dr. Coleman and George Spencer. Visited by George Merritt – Sanitary Agent for State of Ind – Came down on Steamer "Capitola" and going to Vicksburg. On 27th ult- died Martin Shank Private Co H. of typhoid fever. Monthly Report made up and forwarded to H. E. Ellis surgeon of 43rd Ind and Medical Director of portion of 13th Division left at Helena. Rec'd two Monticello papers from Jno. Dixon.

NOTES FOR March 1

Proff. Hibbin: Henry B. Hibbin, Chaplain, 11th Indiana. Residence: Bloomington, Indiana. Date of muster: 3 August 1861.

sanitary agent: Please see entry for March 11 – Sanitary commission.

Capitola: a side-wheel packet built at Wheeling, Virginia in 1860. The U.S. government chartered it for most of the war.[14]

Martin Shank, Pvt., Co. H. Residence: Pulaskiville, Indiana. Date of muster: 5 November 1861. Died at Helena, Arkansas 22 February 1863 of typhoid fever.

H. E. Ellis: Hamilton E. Ellis, Surgeon 43rd Indiana. Residence: Greencastle, Indiana. Date of commission and muster: 9 October 1862. Resigned: 18 June 1863.

March 4.

Yesterday returned from the Regt several sick men and this morning sent back about 50 convalescents under charge of Lt Andrew Co. A. Regt. when last heard from were in Coldwater River, having passed through Moon Lake. Weather warm and pleasant. One year ago to-day was in Nashville, Tennessee. Arrived there on 26th of February just two days after its surrender to Federals. Staid there till about the 8th. Had been left at Cp. Wickliffe, Ky in charge of our sick and started on search of Regt 17th of Feby, found it one month afterwards at New Madrid, Missouri. Our Reg't remained there till after the fight then moved down to Riddle's Point.

NOTES FOR March 4

Lt. Andrew: William A. Andrews, Second Lieutenant, Co. A. Residence: Delphi, Indiana. Enlisted in Company A, 1 November 1861. Date of commission and muster: 20 October 1862. Died 22 May 1863 of wounds sustained at Champion Hill.

New Madrid: Missouri town that suffered a devastating earthquake in 1811 and where (Union) Major General John Pope, Commanding the Army of Mississippi, scored a victory against the Confederates at Fort Thompson on 13 March 1862. New Madrid sits at the middle of a horseshoe bend on the Mississippi River.

Riddle's Point: A point on the Missouri shore of the

Mississippi about fifteen miles downstream from New Madrid opposite Tiptonville, Tennessee where the Indiana 46th and three other regiments constructed a battery.

Helena, Ark's.
March 10, 1863.

Commenced raining last night and been raining ever since. Fair prospect for a long wet spell. Rec'd a letter from Ret. to-day giving the unwelcome news of Dr. Fleming. Think I shall not reply although the third I have rec'd from that service. Three days since returned George Spencer 1st Lt. Co:E. Had been absent since last October. Resignation not accepted. Regt still down the Yazoo Pass. Boats returning from there show they have been much damaged by their trip – chimneys knocked down, wheelhouses torn off rudders lost, and every conceivable injury rec'd from trees, and boughs of trees, snags too. Two days since I was appointed one of a committee to examine all the sick of the division and designate who should go to Gen. Hospital and who were able to join their commands. Dr. Smith Surgeon of the 35th Missouri, Dr Miller of the 28th Wis. Vols. and myself were the committee. After two days' hard labor we finished and made report this morning. Number of division (composed of 9 Regt's and one Battery) to go to Gen. Hosptl numbered 586. To join command 601. Dr. Smith resident of St Louis. Dr. Miller originally from New York City. Many of the class marked for Reg. got on board Hosptl Boat. Consequently sick of our Regt and those of two other Regts' did not get off. Do not know when they will go. Rec'd copy of Hon David Turpie's speech in Senate.

NOTES FOR March 10

Ret.: Underhill's writing is clear here, but what he is referring to is not evident.

"unwelcome news of Dr. Fleming:" (Please see February 7 note.) Fleming appears to have been living in Monticello at this time. Dr. Robert Spencer, one of their teachers at the Cincinnati

College of Medicine and Surgery and a resident of Monticello, had become Surgeon of the Indiana 73rd Infantry. The Indiana Adjutant General's report shows Spencer, by then age 50, as having resigned 21 January 1863. According to an account by his son, he died on February 24, 1864 as a result of disease contracted during the war. Conceivably he resigned for health reasons and that may be the unwelcome news Fleming refers to.

"the third I have received from that service:" The word *service* is hard to decipher and could be *source*.

Dr. Smith: Thomas Smith, Surgeon, 33rd Missouri Infantry. Date of commission and rank: 12 August 1862. Resigned 2 November 1863. Underhill's writing is clear in showing him in the 35th, but the Missouri Adjutant General's Report shows him with the 33rd.

Dr. Miller: Daniel M. Miller, Second Assistant Surgeon, 28th Wisconsin Infantry. Date of commission and rank: 11 September 1862. Upon the dismissal of Lewis K. Hawes, he was promoted 18 November 1863 to First Assistant Surgeon.

Hon. David Turpie: born 8 July 1829, died at Indianapolis 21 April 1909. A Democratic politician and judge who graduated from Kenyon College in 1848, he served as an Indiana state representative, served with the 13th Regiment of the Indiana Volunteers, and at the time of this entry was a U.S. Senator. He later served as a judge and in 1896 was Chair of the Democratic National Convention.

Helena Arks
March 11, 1863.

Unexpectedly weather cleared up last night. To-day a cloudless sky bends over us. Rec'd a call from Sanitary commission on their return from Vicksburg on Steamer Capitola. News from below favorable. More troops going by this evening from Memphis.

NOTES FOR March 11

Sanitary commission: At the outbreak of the war, a number of volunteer groups sprang up to assist soldiers in various ways. Before long, clergy, prominent physicians and others were drawn in and the United States Sanitary Commission became a quasi-official group, with representatives in camps, forts, hospitals, transports, and so on, to ensure clean conditions and to provide relief to the sick and wounded. Their efforts did much to ensure the well-being of the troops. Its first chief executive officer was the famous landscape architect, Frederick Law Olmsted.

March 14

Weather been exceedingly pleasant since the 10th inst. On the 12th was surprised by a call from Dr. Asa Coleman, brother to the Surg. Returned to Memphis this evening. He is now connected with Sanitary commission. Yesterday made a Surgeon's Certificate, for Dr. Ellis Surgeon 43rd, for leave of absence. To-day unexpectedly rec'd note from my old friend and college mate Jno. A. McKee member Co: K. 74th Ohio Regt – now at Murfreesboro Tenn – Wrote letter to-day to Jno Dixon.

NOTES FOR March 14
Dr. Asa Coleman: Residence: Logansport, Indiana. Commissioned 14 May 1862, he had been a pro tem assistant surgeon with the Indiana 46th. He resigned 26 December 1862.

Sabbath Eve – March 15

Attended divine service at Fort Curtis. Heard a good address from our Chaplain Rev. Robb. Col. Bussey of Iowa also made an excellent patriotic address. He is a tall fine looking gentleman about six feet high, dark hair large whiskers all over his face, but not so dark as his hair – complexion pale – a keen eye – pleasant expression of countenance of spare form – altogether forming a gentleman of apparently about 33 years of age and one who would be noticed in a large crowd as above the mediocrity. He is a pleasant and expressive speaker enunciation excellent – was attended by two ladies. He was followed by Gen Prentiss the Commander of the District. The general is a gentleman of perhaps fifty years though he looks older than he really is. His form is neat and well built – height about 5 feet 8 ½ – a fine head for a phrenologist – hair streaked with gray and closely cut – skin rather dark. His remarks were to the point and made some good hits. Spoke of his capture at Shiloh and treatment he suffered. Altogether he made a favorable impression – about one thousand persons present. A few regiments came down the river to-day. Some of their boys leaving the boats became intoxicated and a melee ensued in which some of the Provost guards wounded two of the rioters – one dangerously. Boats then crossed to the opposite side of river — Wrote letter to David Wallace, also Jno. McKee, and a short note to Linnie J_____ Weather warm and pleasant.

NOTES FOR March 15

Col. Bussey of Iowa: Cyrus Bussey (1833-1915). He was born in Ohio, raised in Indiana, and settled in Iowa in 1855. He was a member of the state legislature and delegate to the convention that nominated Stephen Douglas in 1860. He had numerous assignments. On this date he was commanding the 2nd Brigade, 2nd Division, Cavalry, 13th Corps, Army of the Tennessee. He later became a brigadier general and after the war became a Republican and was active in Louisiana politics.[15]

Gen Prentiss: See notes for October 30 and February 19. General Prentiss's division was taken by surprise when the Confederates attacked at Shiloh. By early afternoon he was holding a critical position along a lane which Grant had ordered him to hold at any cost. After withstanding wave after wave of attacks and vastly outnumbered, Prentiss was finally overcome late in the afternoon and surrendered his forces, at which time he was taken prisoner.

David Wallace: Most likely David Wallace who appears in the 1860 Guernsey County, Ohio census as a farmer, 56, or his son, David H., listed as 16.

Helena, Ark's.
Saturday Morn March 21 –

Early part of present week returned Dr. Horace Coleman. Next morning started in company with all the Surgeons of Division remaining here to join the Division. Our division had proceeded as far as Greenwood at the mouth of the Tallahatchie River. There the Tallahatchie and Yallabusha unite to form the Yazoo distant from here by water about 200 miles. Rebels have fortifications there and some fighting has been going on. News rec'd that Stewart of Co: B. was mortally wounded, Rogers of the same Co: severely wounded – Col. Bringhurst struck with piece of shell on the arm injured but little. But two surgeons Dr. Varny and myself are left here in care of the sick of the division. Day before yesterday Surg Jessup 24th Ind – Surg McClure and myself were appointed by order of Gen Prentiss a Medical Board to examine into the physical health of Asst. Surg. Crosby of 47th Ind who neglected, alleging ill health as an excuse, to join regiment as ordered. Been reading for a few days a work of fiction entitled "John Halifax" by Miss Mulock. Has been praised much by many good critics, but I am not so highly pleased with it as I had anticipated. The story ends well, however, which is saying a great deal for it. Principal Characters John Halifax, Abel Fletcher, Phinias Fletcher, Miss Ursula March, Lady Caroline Brithwood, Earl of Luxmore, Lord Ravenel, Guy Halifax, Edwin Halifax, Miss Louise D'Argent, Miss Maud Halifax, and Miss Grace Oldtower. Rec'd letter from home day before yesterday – all well – written by M___S_____. Private Michael Blue Co:F. died 19th inst of typhoid fever. Must go to breakfast.

NOTES FOR March 21

Stewart: Samuel Stewart, Pvt., Co. B. Residence: New Waverly, Indiana. Date of muster 5 November 1861. Underhill's report of Stewart's being mortally wounded was incorrect. He was shot through the groin at Fort Pemberton, Mississippi on 11 March 1863 and was transferred to the Invalid Corps 2 January 1864 and mustered out from that organization.

Rogers: Theophilus P. Rodgers. Enlisted 5 November 1861.

Rodgers was shot in the leg. He was commissioned first lieutenant 27 December 1864 and mustered out with the regiment.

Dr. Varny: Possibly Royal W. Varney, Assistant Surgeon from April 1863 in the Ohio 31st Infantry. Mustered out 20 July 1865. The Ohio 31st was not at Helena on March 21 but Varney might have served in another unit prior to joining the 31st or have been on temporary duty.

Surg. McClure: Samuel M. McClure, Assistant Surgeon, Indiana 37th. Residence: Westport, Indiana. Date of commission and muster: 18 November 1862. Resigned 15 February 1864.

Asst. Surg. Crosby: Thomas Crosby, Assistant Surgeon, Indiana 47th. Residence: Bluffton, Indiana. Date of commission: 25 November 1862. Date of muster: 25 December 1862. Mustered out 21 December 1864 when term expired.

John Halifax, Gentleman was written by Dinah Maria Mulock Craik (1826-1887), an English novelist born in Staffordshire who later moved to London and eventually to Kent. The title page merely says "by the author of" "Olive," "The Ogilvies," "Agatha's Husband," "Avillion," "The Head of the Family," "Nothing New," "A Hero, and Other Tales, &c." *John Halifax, Gentleman* (1856) was her most successful work. The story is told in a first person narrative by Phineas Fletcher, a very sickly man whose father, Abel Fletcher, a Quaker, takes in a destitute boy named John Halifax as an apprentice in his tan yard and gives him a good start in life. Phineas and John are like brothers, and since Phineas never marries or carries on the father's affairs, John takes over, and after Abel Fletcher's death, Phineas lives with John and his family. The story then traces the ascent in early 19th century British society of John Halifax and his wife, Ursula March, and their children, as he prospers in business and makes much money by converting a mill from water to steam power. As a man of trade with humble beginnings, he is resented by some of the gentry and titled folk but finally shows himself morally superior to many with his ethical business behavior and happy marriage. In places the story is saccharine, but compared with *The Count of Paris*, it is an engaging novel.

M__S___: an unknown reference.

Michael Blue Co. F: In the *History of the Forty-Sixth Regiment*

Indiana Volunteer Infantry, Blue is shown as a private and a detailed musician who died at Helena, Arkansas, 25 December 1862. This date of death appears incorrect.

March 26, 1863.

Weather pleasant to-day – quite cool last night – Monday and Tuesday rainy and cold. Day before yesterday returned from the Regt. Lieut. George W. Spencer came to take all men able for duty sent down 40 – old soldiers generally. Wrote a long letter home few days ago. Also rec'd one from George T. Wilson resident of Burnettsville Somerset County Maryland – represents my friend Elijah Ward as going Secesh. Attended church in the Fort last Sabbath. Among other addresses a very pleasant one was made by Col. Cameron of 34th Indiana. This week been reading Dickens' "Great Expectations." Finished it to-day and much pleased with it. Principal Characters Mr. Pip, Joe Gargery and wife, also Biddy afterwards his second wife – Estella, the protege of old Miss Havisham – Mr. Pumblechook – Mr. Wopsle Clerk at church – Mr. Jaggers the lawyer, Mr. Wemmick his clerk – Herbert – Pip's friend and companion. The two convicts Abel Magwitch also Compey, and Oslick. The upshot of the whole is that Pip never realizes his expectations – Miss Havisham dies – Miss Estella marries a drone by the name of Drummle much to the disgust of Pip who passionately loved her. It turns out that Estella is daughter of Magwitch the convict by a gipsy afterward housekeeper to Mr. Jaggers. Herbert marries a nice little girl by the name of Miss Clara Barley. Wemmick very unostentatiously weds Miss Skiffins. Pip finally goes in partnership, with his friend Herbert going to the East after first clerking with him for some time – and is never married, but returns to visit Joe Gargery where his earliest days were past – – – A good story and having read it don't see where or how it would be improved. Wright Nield, Private Co D – had his arm blown off by a cannon ball at Greenwood Miss. Arm afterwards amputated by Dr. Dicken Brigade Surgeon and subject died in a few days.

NOTES FOR March 26

Elijah Ward: Elijah Smith Ward, Jr. (1836-1921). A childhood friend and contemporary of Underhill's from Quindocqua, Maryland. Since Confederate units could not be raised in Maryland, Ward joined Capt. Dent's Battery, Light Artillery, a unit raised directly by the CSA. Underhill was a little out of date: Ward was enlisted as a private at Pensacola by Capt. F. H. Robertson 21 December 1861 for the duration of the war. He was shown as absent on the 1 July - 31 August 1862 muster roll because of being a nurse in a hospital. Ward deserted while on furlough 24 October 1863 but returned to duty to show up as present on the 31 October - 31 December 1863 muster roll. He married Caroline B. Adams. Ward is buried in St. Paul's Cemetery, Marion, Maryland.

Wright L. Nield, Pvt., Co. D. Wounded at Fort Pemberton, Mississippi, 19 March 1863. Nield was trying to spot a rebel gun that was firing at a working squad. He saw the gun fire but could not get down in time and had an arm shot off. He died of his wounds.

Dr. Dicken: James L. Dicken, Surgeon, 47th Indiana. Residence: Wabash, Indiana. Date of commission: 21 October 1861. Date of muster: 13 December 1861. Mustered out with the regiment.

March 31, 1863

Corporal John Chamberlain discharged yesterday – his father had come for him. Weather been quite cold for two or three days – high winds – moderating a little to-day. Made up to day Monthly Report and Return Medical Officers and forwarded directly to Medical Director Hammond. Rec'd copy Guernsey Times to-day. Also note from Miss S. P. of Mansfield. Think I shall not reply. Sick came up from the Pass. Report our regiment at Greenwood and fight imminent. Was quite sick yesterday suffering from nervous headache.

NOTES FOR March 31
John Chamberlain: Cpl. Co., H. Residence: Winamac, Indiana. Date of muster: 5 November 1861. Discharged 7 April 1863.

Guernsey Times: a newspaper printed at Cambridge, Ohio.

Miss S. P.: Her identity is unknown but possibly she may have been someone Underhill knew at Madison College.

April 2 – 1863.

Weather fine and pleasant for last few days. Wrote letter to Jno. Dixon. Made up Quarterly Requisition. Heard our division was on their route back from Greenwood – leaving Quimby's brigade there also some gunboats. Haines Bluff evacuated few days ago. This is a beautiful calm moonlight night – just been listening to some good instrumental music – guitar, two violins and flute – Taps! and I'll retire to rest.

NOTES FOR April 2
Greenwood: The county seat of Leflore County, Mississippi, about ninety miles north northeast of Vicksburg.

Haines Bluff: Sometimes spelled Haynes Bluff, it was on the east side of the Yazoo River about ten or twelve miles above the mouth of the Yazoo. The Confederates had fortified it heavily.

Quimby: (Union) Brigadier General Isaac Ferdinand Quinby (1821-1891). A native of New Jersey, he graduated from West Point in 1843 and returned there to teach. He left a professorship at the University of Rochester, New York to enter the war. In March 1862 he became a brigadier general of volunteers. At the time Underhill writes of him, he was commanding the 7th Division, 17th Corps, Army of the Tennessee, and participated in operations against Corinth and later was on the Yazoo Pass expedition. During the Vicksburg campaign he was ill but fought at Champion Hill, Big Black River, and in the May assault against Vicksburg. In June 1863 he had to give up his command.[16]

Helena Arkansas
April 4- 1863

Rec'd today a poem "The Wounded Soldier" composed by my old college mate J. A. McKee Co K 74th Reg. O. Vol. Inf. It was written after the battle of Stone's River in which engagement he participated. To-day the three years for which I volunteered are half expired. The next 18 months will soon pass away. Date of the commission of the first officers was Oct -4- 1861, making to-day eighteen months our Regt has been in service.

NOTES FOR April 4
Stone's River: see January 10 entry for Murfreesboro.

Sabbath Eve April 5th

Attended Divine Service to-day in the fort to-day. Sermon preached by an Iowa Chaplain. Then followed an effective address from Lieut. Col. Wood of First Indiana Cavalry – also a speech by Col. McGill of 29th Wisconsin volunteers. Exercises by a masterly address from Gen. Prentiss – now a Major General. He spoke of his birth and parentage, reviewed his sufferings from the treatment of Rebels while a captive, and concluded by a few words of timely and good advice to his soldiers and officers. He was cheered almost continually throughout his remarks. Would that all our Generals were like him ——Last night died Private John Warwick: Co: G. Weather fine and pleasant. To-morrow a force of two thousand go on an expedition up St. Francis River under command of Brig. Gen. Willis A. Gorman.

NOTES FOR April 5
St. Francis River: A river in Arkansas north of Helena emptying into the L'Anguille River in Lee County.

Col. Wood: William F. Wood. Residence: Rockport, Indiana. Date of commission and muster: 7 November 1861. Resigned 2 April 1863 to become colonel of a newly-formed black regiment.

Col. McGill 29th Wisc.: The Wisconsin Adjutant General's report lists both in 1862 and 1864 Colonel Charles R. Gill as colonel of the 29th Wisconsin with a date of rank and date of commission of 30 August 1862.

Pvt. John W. Warwick, Co. G: Date of muster 5 November 1861.

Tuesday Morning April 7, 1863.

Yesterday arrived L. Thomas Adjutant General of the U.S. Army. He comes for the purpose of arranging for the recruiting at this place of negroes. Word was dispatched to the different regts. that he would speak in the fort at three o'clock. Accordingly before that hour the fort was filled with soldiers impatiently awaiting the announcement of the General. Not less than 4,000 were in the fort. It will be remembered that a great portion of the army at Helena are temporarily absent – Gen Ross's division being down the Yazoo Pass – and Gen. W. A. Gorman being up the St. Francis River——Gen. Thomas briefly made known the purpose for which he was visiting the different portions of the Army. He was enthusiastically cheered at almost every sentence of his short address. The General is apparently about sixty years of age, but years sit lightly on him. He is of fine athletic form – full six feet high well muscled and straight as an arrow. His hair is perfectly white and he is altogether the very personification of a <u>venerable</u> hero. His short speech was followed by a few remarks from Major General Prentiss who was almost continually cheered. Brig. Gen. Alvin P. Hovey followed in a few brilliant and eloquent words. Gen. Hovey is a young man of prepossessing and romantic appearance. A little above the medium size, handsome features, a head the beau-ideal of the phrenologist. He is a statesman, scholar, soldier, and gentleman, a man destined to rise to yet greater fame. No man is more popular with his men than Gen. A. P. Hovey with his division. Next followed Major General Washburne who was well received and spoke many words of good cheer. He is a large man weighing perhaps two hundred. Short neck, full face, not very expressive, hair flaxen and slightly bald. He is well liked by his men.

Hon. Mr. Mitchell Member Congress from Indiana also spoke – had been on a visit to army at Vicksburg. He is no doubt an able, sound man, and good thinker but no speaker. He is a gentleman of perhaps 55 years of age, with good head, smooth, broad face – and a countenance beaming with benignity and honest integrity. Col. Cameron 34th Ind – Col Bussey of some Iowa Regt – also Col McGill of 29th Wisconsin afterwards addressed the assemblage. Capt Cameron of 9th Ill. Cavalry and Provost Marshal at this place addressed the audience eloquently. A few ladies, principally officers' wives, graced the meeting with their presence. The enthusiasm of the army has never been as great since we left Indiana as it has been for the last month.

Helena, Arks.
Tuesday Evening April 7.

Rec'd letter to-day from my old friend "chum," and college mate – Jno. A. McKee. 9th I'll. Cavalry leave for Memphis to-day. Weather very pleasant.

NOTES FOR April 7

L. Thomas Adjutant General of the U.S. Army: Brigadier General Lorenzo Thomas (1804-1875) graduated from West Point in 1823. When his official report on the activities of John C. Frémont in Missouri led to Frémont's removal, Thomas made enemies, including Edwin Stanton, later Secretary of War. Lincoln protected Thomas who was eventually assigned to recruiting black troops in the West. He was later brevetted major general and continued as Adjutant General until his retirement in 1869.[17]

Mr. Mitchell, Member of Congress, Indiana: William Mitchell, born in 1808 in Montgomery County, New York, moved to Indiana in 1836 and built a log cabin at Kendalville, which was wilderness at the time. He was elected to the Indiana legislature in 1842 and in 1860 was elected to Congress. He was a strong Union supporter and in 1863 established the First National Bank of Kendalville and served as its president until he died, which would have been before 1875.[18]

Capt. Cameron, 9th Illinois Cavalry: Most likely Charles S. Cameron, discharged 31 December 1863.

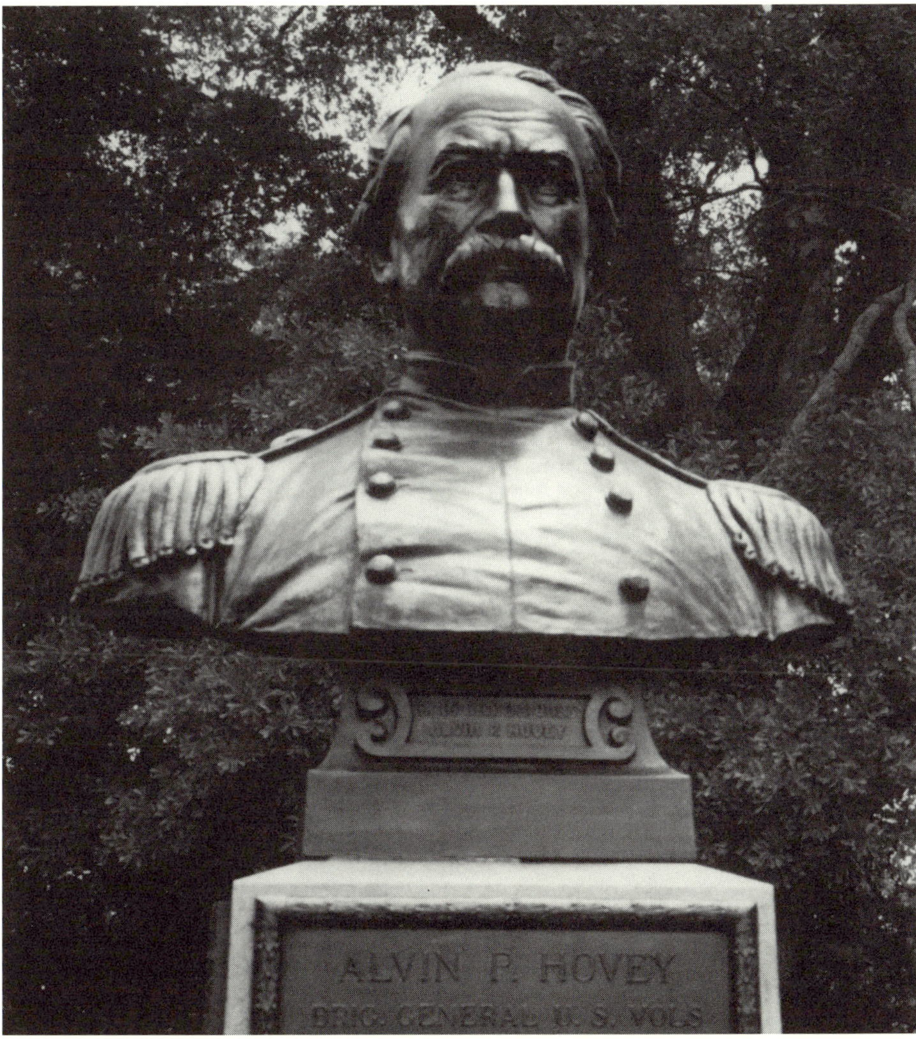

"No man is more popular with his men than Gen. A.P. Hovey," Underhill observes in his diary on 7 April 1863, writing of the Indiana native who was then commanding Union troops in eastern Arkansas. Soon, Hovey would lead Underhill and others south to take part in the Vicksburg Campaign. On May 16th, Underhill and the rest of Hovey's troops would have a central but costly role in the Battle of Champion Hill, about half way between Jackson and Vicksburg. They would then move on to Vicksburg. Today a bust of Hovey stands at the Vicksburg Military Park, inscribed: "ALVIN P. HOVEY/ BRIG. GENERAL OF U.S. VOLS/ COMMANDING 12TH DIVISION/ THIRTEENTH ARMY CORPS."

Thursday Evening April 9, 1863

Yesterday afternoon returned the regt. from Yazoo Pass Expedition. Since they left they have lost killed two – wounded six and drowned one. Expedition a failure. Rumored that we leave for Vicksburg to-morrow. Regt. still lying on boat. Yesterday I met my fellow medical student Killian whom I had not seen before since February 1861. Is now Hospital Steward 1st Ind. Cav. Rec'd also to-day a letter from Linnie first since last winter – brother died at Nashville in Hospital. Wrote yesterday to Jno. A McKee, Murfreesboro. A contraband regiment is being raised here – Lt. Col. Wood 1st Indiana Cav. is Col – Capt Campbell 34th Ind–Lt. Col. and Capt Burson of 46th Major. Weather warm.

NOTES FOR April 9

Killian, Hosp. Steward 1st Ind. Cavalry: Probably John L. Killian, listed in the Indiana Adjutant General's Report as a recruit, from Vandenburg County. Date of muster: 15 October 1862. Although Underhill and Killian may have known each other in Cincinnati as medical students, Killian does not appear in any roster at the Cincinnati College of Medicine and Surgery, the Medical College of Ohio, or the Eclectic Medical Institute.

contraband: "Contraband" was the term given to slaves who had escaped from their masters. An all-black unit was being formed here.

Capt. Campbell: James W. Campbell, Co. B, Indiana 34th. Date of commission: 16 September 1861. Date of muster: 30 September 1861. Promoted to lieutenant colonel, 1st Arkansas Colored Regiment, 21 April 1863.

Captain Burson: George W. Burson, First Lieutenant, Co. H, 46th Indiana. Residence: Winamac. Date of commission: 4 October 1861. Date of muster: 5 November 1861. Promoted to captain. Date of commission 29 May 1862.

On Board Steamer Volunteer
Friday Night April 10.

Lying on boat to night everything moved down to-day. Regt paid off by Maj Mitchell. Perhaps move down the river to-morrow.

NOTES FOR April 10

Volunteer: a stern-wheel packet built at Monongahela, Pennsylvania in 1862 and chartered to the government at $150 per day. The *Volunteer* had been used for the Yazoo Pass expedition. According to the *History of the Forty-Sixth Regiment Indiana Volunteer Infantry*, it was a very handsome new boat, fresh from Pittsburgh. After the expedition, it was an utter mess. Smokestacks had been knocked down and upper works destroyed.[19]

Maj. Mitchell: Not shown in the roster of the 46th. A James F. Mitchell of Company H is shown as promoted to captain but there is no evidence in the *History of the Forty-Sixth Regiment Indiana Volunteer Infantry* of his having been promoted to major.

On Board Volunteer
Sabbath morn April 12.

Lying up to shore on Arkansas side 7 miles below Helena. Arrived here yesterday afternoon and waiting to collect the fleet. Have been transferred to Gen. Hovey's division again and are in the Brigade commanded by Brevet Brig. Gen'l. McGinnis of 11th Ind. Our division and a portion of Gen. Quimby's constitute the forces moving down the river. Rained last night but is clear and beautiful this morning. Oh – what a lovely Sabbath morn! But "war knows no Sabbath." Weather too warm to be comfortable.

Sunday Evening

Got under way half past eleven o'clock A.M. Made good time all day. Passed Napoleon just before sunset town almost entirely deserted. Arkansas River empties into Mississippi at that point. Only building noticed especially at Napoleon was a large three story building – The Marine Hospital just below the junction of the rivers.

NOTES FOR April 12
Brevet Brig. Gen. McGinnis: George Francis McGinnis (1826-1910). Born in Boston, he was a hatter in Indiana. He served in the Mexican War. Residence: Indianapolis, Indiana. Date of commission and muster as colonel: 3 September 1861. Promoted to (Union) brigadier general 29 November 1862. He was a friend of Lew Wallace and John McClernand and for that reason may have been given a series of minor commands. He was at Fort Donelson, Shiloh, the advance to Corinth, the Yazoo Pass expedition, and in the Vicksburg campaign, and later went with the 13th Corps to the Gulf. He mustered out in August 1865.[20]

On Steamer Volunteer
Monday April 13th 1863.

Last night kept under way nearly all night. Lay up two or three hours in latter part of night. This forenoon we are passing camps at Lake Providence. Rainy morning. One year ago this morning we left Tiptonville Tennessee under command of Gen. Pope and steamed down to Fort Pillow which we reached that afternoon. Then Pope could have moved on to New Orleans, but he was ordered to Shiloh and our regt lay off Fort Pillow till it was evacuated by the Secesh. We entered it on the 4th of June. We are one year too late in our attempts to take Vicksburg. This morning died suddenly Jacob Quinn private Co. F.

Milliken's Bend Louisiana
Monday Night April 13.

To-night we are lying tied up to shore. To-morrow we make a land march but where we know not yet. Wrote a note home.

NOTES FOR April 13

Lake Providence: a lake in northeast Louisiana at the head of the Tensas River. Grant had a plan to cut a channel from the Mississippi into the lake, thereby getting a water route south through the Tensas and several other rivers that would rejoin the Mississippi south of Natchez, thus getting around Vicksburg. This plan was never completed.

Tiptonville, Tennessee: in northwest Tennessee close to the Mississippi River and about twenty miles south of New Madrid, Missouri but only about five miles from Island No. 10.

Fort Pillow: Fort Pillow lay on the Tennessee shore of the Mississippi, about seventy miles north of Memphis. It sat on bluffs seventy-five to one hundred feet high, and because of bends in the river, had a commanding view for several miles both up and downstream. Held by the Confederates, it had to be taken. After naval action on 17 April 1862 and again on May 10, it was abandoned by the Confederates June 4 after they had suffered defeats elsewhere in Tennessee and were threatened with being virtually cut off.

Pope: (Union) Major General John Pope (1822-1892) commanded the Army of the Mississippi and had led the attack on New Madrid and Island No. 10.

Jacob Quinn private Co. F.: Quinn is listed in the *History of the Forty-Sixth Regiment Indiana Volunteer Infantry* and in the Indiana Adjutant General's Report as a corporal. Residence: Camden, Indiana. He died at Milliken's Bend, Louisiana, 15 April 1863. Date of muster: 14 November 1861.

Richmond, Parish Madison, Louisiana
Thursday Evening, April 16, 1863

Did not march next day after writing last paragraph. Left Millikens Bend, this morning en route for Carthage. Distance marched 12 miles to-day 18 to Carthage from here. Richmond small village population perhaps 100. Marched over some very fine plantations. Stopped at a country mansion hospitably treated. Visited a signal station commanded by Lt Fisher 34th Ind.

NOTES FOR April 16
Milliken's Bend: A Federal camp on the Louisiana shore of the Mississippi, roughly twenty-five miles by water above Vicksburg. It had perhaps five hundred people and several churches. Because of changes in the river it no longer exists.

Carthage: A modern map does not show this. A period map shows a town of New Carthage, on the Louisiana shore about twenty miles south of Vicksburg. The plantation of Jefferson Davis lay directly across the river on the Mississippi shore.

Richmond: A little inland town, shown on a period map about fifteen miles southwest of Milliken's Bend. Richmond would have been part way between Milliken's Bend and New Carthage, which lay about twelve miles southeast.

Lt. Fisher: Hiram G. Fisher, First Lieutenant, 34th Indiana. Residence: Fishersburg, Indiana. Date of commission: 16 September 1861. Date of muster: 10 October 1861. Resigned 14 July 1863.

Saturday morning April 18.

No march to-day – are camping 12 miles from Richmond and about 6 from Carthage. Beautiful camping ground. Yesterday passed the plantation of Gen. Holmes. So far as we have marched the country is a perfect paradise of a place. Several cotton gins burned yesterday and other buildings wantonly destroyed. We camp without tents, our tents baggage etc. being left on trans-

port Cheeseman. Slept under the stars last two nights. Gen. Smith's division is encamped near us. Gen Osterhaus' a little further along.

NOTES FOR April 18

Gen. Holmes: (Confederate) Lieutenant General Theophilus Hunter Holmes, 1804-1880. A North Carolina-born graduate of West Point in 1829, he had served in the Mexican War and was the Confederate commander in Arkansas who led the unsuccessful attack on Fort Curtis in July 1863. Hearing loss affected his performance and he was eased out of any important position.[21]

Gen. Smith: (Union) Brigadier General Andrew Jackson Smith (1815-1897) was a career Army officer, native of Pennsylvania and Class of 1838 at West Point. From 12 January to 7 August 1863, he was commanding the 10th Division, 13th Corps, Army of the Tennessee. He was with Sherman at Chickasaw Bayou, McClernand at Arkansas Post, Grant at Vicksburg, and Nathaniel P. Banks on the Red River Campaign.[22]

Sabbath Eve April 19.

Wrote two letters to-day one to Dr. W. S. Haymond, Monticello, Ind, and one to J. A. McKee. Yesterday wrote one to Linnie. Rained very heavily last night clear and pleasant to-day. News first rec'd of capture of Charleston – by Admiral Dupont and Gen. Hunter considered extremely doubtful.

Tuesday Eve. April 21, 1863

This morning regt. and division took up their line of march for Carthage. I am left to look after a few sick and clean up things generally. Raining heavy this morning. Been rather unwell since we came here – suffering from nervous debility.

Friday, April 24, 1863.

Yesterday afternoon reached regiment which is camped about three miles below Carthage and close to the Roundaway Bayou. We are now bridging the bayou and will cross to the Mississippi shore distant about 2 ½ miles. There we will go on board transports but for what purpose is not known. Night before last quite a number of transports ran the Rebel blockade and are now below Vicksburg. One or two were destroyed. Wrote a letter home to-day.

NOTES FOR April 24
Because of problems moving enough supplies overland, six more steamers, loaded with supplies and towing a dozen barges carrying rations, ran the batteries on the night of April 22.

Saturday morning, April 25.

Pleasant morning – days a little warm. Thermometer reaches 90° in the afternoon. Wrote to George T. Wilson this morning. The boats that ran the blockade the last night were the "Empire City," "Moderator," "Anglo-Saxon," and "J. W. Cheeseman." The "Tigress" in making the attempt was almost destroyed. The loss was 22 killed and wounded. The "Henry Clay" was not burned as reported a few nights ago in her attempt to run the blockade.

NOTES FOR April 25
Empire City: a stern-wheel packet built at California, Pennsylvania in 1854 and used from 1862-1865 as a transport.[23]

Moderator: a stern-wheel packet built at Brownsville, Pennsylvania in 1856. A week after this entry she sank the *Horizon* in a collision at Grand Gulf.[24]

Anglo-Saxon: a side-wheel packet built at Beaver County, Pennsylvania in 1857 which had seen government service in the Tennessee River campaign.[25]

J. W. Cheesman: a stern-wheel packet built at Cincinnati in 1856 and under contract to the U.S. government during the war.

Earlier in April, the captain was killed on board by a Confederate on the shore of the Yazoo River. Underhill spells her name *Cheeseman*.[26]

Tigress: a side-wheel packet built at Cincinnati in 1858. It helped rescue survivors after the *Eugene* was wrecked at Osceola (see Nov. 16 entry) and was lost after being hit running the Vicksburg batteries. The *J. W. Cheesman* rescued the entire crew with no loss of life.[27]

Henry Clay: a side-wheel packet built at McKeesport, Pennsylvania in 1858. She was burned and lost running the Vicksburg batteries, contrary to Underhill's report.[28]

Sabbath Eve April 26th

Bridges over different bayous are finished and we cross to morrow. To-day Dr. Coleman rejoined reg't. Day quite pleasant.

Monday Evening

This evening finds us encamped near the bank of the Mississippi. It is expected that we will cross either to night or to-morrow. If we do a bloody fight will in all probability take place. Four divisions of us are now here. Been raining nearly all day.

Wednesday 11 o'clock A.M.
near Grand Gulf Mississippi

Yesterday we embarked on Forest Queen and came down arriving here before daylight this morning. We are nearly 4 miles distant lying on our transport watching the fight between the enemys batteries and our gunboats. The ball opened at 8 o'clock this morning and has continued with little intermission till present time. If the batteries are silenced we will land our troops from the transports. Four divisions are here Gens Grant, McPherson, McClernand – also Adjutant Gen Thomas and Gov. Yates of Illinois. Yesterday rec'd letter from Dr. Fleming one also from home. Wrote two notes one home and one to Dr. McPherson.

NOTES FOR April 29
Forest Queen: a side-wheel packet built at Madison, Indiana in 1858 that saw much service during the war.[29]

Grand Gulf: a town on the Mississippi shore about eight miles north of Bruinsburg and perhaps forty miles south of Vicksburg by water.

Gen. McPherson: (Union) Major General James Birdseye McPherson (1828-1864). Ohio born, he was the head of his class at West Point in 1853. An engineer, he taught at West Point and worked on both coasts as an engineer. He served for a time as an aide to General Halleck and later became Grant's engineering chief. Commander of the Seventeenth Corps under Grant, he saw action in the Vicksburg campaign and was later killed in action at Decatur, Georgia in July 1864.[30]

Gen. McClernand: (Union) Major General John A. McClernand (1816-1900) relieved Sherman after the Chickasaw Bayou attack, captured Arkansas Post, and commanded a corps at Vicksburg. He appears to have been a brilliant but egotistical man who grated on people and whose rather bizarre behavior at Vicksburg called his judgment into question. Grant relieved him of command at Vicksburg and assigned Major General Ord in his place.

Adjutant General Thomas: see note for April 7.

Gov. Yates of Ilinois: Richard Yates, 1818-1873. He was a staunch Republican and governor of Illinois 1861-1865. He served in the U.S. Senate from 1865-1871.

Thursday Evening April 30

This evening finds us camped a few miles below in the rear of Grand Gulf. Bombardment was kept up yesterday till 2 o'clock P.M. making a six hour fight. Of the 8 Rebel batteries two could not be silenced. Troops landed and marched across stinking river below. Transports ran by the batteries without material damage. Heavy bombardment little after dark. Entire loss on gunboats as follows: Benton 7 killed and 12 wounded – Pittsburgh 6 killed and 20 wounded – Tuscumbia 5 killed and 19 wounded – Some reported injured on the other boats. 7 boats engaged – Benton, Pittsburgh, Lafayette, Tuscumbia, Mound City, Louisville, and Carondelet. Our regt crossed this morning on Benton. 4 divisions on this side of river now.

NOTES FOR April 30

Benton: The Benton was originally a snag boat converted to an ironclad in 1861. (A snag boat is a steamboat with apparatus designed to catch debris in the water.) It was twice as large as other ironclads and had been Commodore Foote's flagship. On this crossing the Indiana 46th occupied the gun deck while General Grant and Admiral Porter stood in the wheel house.

Pittsburgh: spelled *Pittsburg* in most references. One of the seven city-class gunboats.

Lafayette: a side-wheeler purchased in St. Louis and under the direction of Navy Commander William Porter converted into an ironclad. It was contracted for by the Army, as were the city-class boats.

Tuscumbia: an ironclad side-wheeler contracted for by the Navy and built by Joseph Brown in Cincinnati. It pounded Vicksburg during the siege. It was a sister ship of the *Indianola* and the *Chillicothe*.

Saturday morning May 2nd–

Day before yesterday marched from the river at 3 P.M. Marched all night and arrived at the outposts of the enemy about daylight. 1st Ind. Battery lost one or two killed and 7 wounded. We took ½ hour's sleep and a little coffee. Carr's division moved on the enemy at 6 o'clock and our division (Gen Hovey's) came up just as they were beginning to give away. At 7 o'clock a terrific fight occurred in which we finally drove the enemy from the field capturing a number of prisoners and two batteries of artillery. Our division was engaged about 8 hours and our brigade 5 hours. Loss of our regt. and division impossible to ascertain as yet. The entire loss, however, is heavy. Rebels fought with the greatest desperation and bravery but we drove them at every point and are now only 2 ½ miles from Port Gibson. Last night we were called up but the alarm was false. Both parties have been reenforced during the last night and the contest may be renewed this morning unless the enemy fall back. Our regt and 24th Ind made the charge and took two batteries, the 46th taking as many prisoners as the regt. numbered.

Port Gibson 11 o'clock

Enemy crossed bayou and in their retreat perhaps they will make a stand this side Black River. They burned the bridge behind them. We are now constructing bridges across the bayou to follow them. Port Gibson a nice town. When citizens at home number perhaps three thousand – county seat of Claiborne County. This morning on march found good many dead Secesh. Genl Tracy reported killed. Our regimental loss was 8 killed 36 wounded 4 to 6 of whom are mortally, many slightly wounded not reported. Distance from here to the point where we marched from on the Mississippi is 18 miles – 17 miles to the Black River 8 miles distant to Grand Gulf.

NOTES FOR May 2

Gen. Carr: (Union) Brigadier General Eugene A. Carr (1830-1910) was born at Concord, NY and graduated from West Point in 1850. He was awarded the Medal of Honor for not leaving the battlefield at Pea Ridge despite being wounded. He was the senior Union commander at the start of the battle for Port Gibson. After the war he earned a reputation as a renowned Indian fighter.

Port Gibson: A town about thirty miles south of Vicksburg by road, several miles inland from the Mississippi River and the seat of Claiborne County.

Gen. Tracy: (Confederate) Brigadier General Edward Dorr

Tracy (1833-1863), whose unit had made a forty-four mile forced march from Vicksburg to confront Grant after the landing at Bruinsburg. He died in the action at Port Gibson. He was born in Georgia but moved to Alabama, becoming a lawyer.[31]

Black River: the Big Black River. River in Mississippi running south southwest in western Mississippi and a few miles east of Vicksburg.

Sunday Eve May 3rd 1863

Left Port Gibson this morning half past six o'clock. Crossed Bayou Pierre on bridge constructed by pioneer corps. Scouted the woods for miles southwest of town. Returned to main road and followed after the army about sundown crossed Tallahatta Creek and camped just by the side – or rather it was the bayou we crossed which is formed by the Tallahatta Creek and South Branch. Distance marched 8 miles besides distance traveled in scouring the country. An attempt was made by the retreating enemy to burn the last bridge, a neat suspension structure, but our advance drove them off in which there was a skirmish. Country through which we have passed since crossing river at Bruinsburg is very hilly.

NOTES FOR May 3

Bruinsburg: the landing point Grant chose for disembarking his troops. Named after Peter Bryan Bruin, it lay south of Vicksburg about forty-five miles on the Mississippi side. Because of the Chickasaw Bayou failure, Grant decided to move his troops south by river to Milliken's Bend, Louisiana and then march them south on the Louisiana side to avoid having to transport them by water past the Vicksburg batteries. The troops were then moved across the river to Bruinsburg in preparation to move north against Vicksburg. Bruinsburg no longer exists.

Monday Night – May 4 –

Moved camp about one mile rested during day – boys were out foraging great portion of the time. Weather warm and dry. Grand Gulf was taken possession of yesterday.

Tuesday May 5, 1863.

Remained here all day waiting for rations – not come yet. Passed the day pleasantly under the shade of spreading beeches and magnolias. A great many magnolias beautify these forests. Some of the largest kind nearly as large as the great oaks that enrich our Northern forests. To-day wrote a note home. Rec'd two letters by mail one from Ross Wallace and one from Linnie. Dr. Coleman and Hospital Steward Doan came up with regt having been back at Gen. Hospital with wounded. Rec'd invoice of medicines.

NOTES FOR May 5
Ross Wallace: R. R. Wallace of the 74th Ohio. Underhill mentions answering this letter on May 8. John A. McKee, a frequent correspondent, was in the same unit.

Hospital Steward Doan: George M. Doane. Enlisted in Company B, 5 November 1861. Commissioned assistant surgeon 1 January 1865 following Underhill's promotion to surgeon after Israel Washburn mustered out. Underhill wrote Governor Morton a warm letter of recommendation for Doane's promotion, calling him "thoroughly loyal, of good morale, and always attentive." Doane mustered out with the regiment 4 September 1865.

Near Rock Springs, Mississippi
Thursday morning May 7

Yesterday morning took up line of march at 5 o'clock, made 8 miles by 9 o'clock and went into camp. Here we will probably remain till we get rations.

Provision is getting scarce and we are compelled to forage. Weather quite cool for season and latitude.

Thursday Evening

Marched this afternoon two miles. Are now camped near the enemy which is reported on this side of Black River – distance to river three miles. We have now come into a region of pines which are now as numerous as magnolias were a few days ago although they are not large. Wrote a letter to Linnie J______.

NOTES FOR May 7
Rock Springs: It should be Rocky Springs. It lies about fifteen miles northeast of Port Gibson, Mississippi.

Friday afternoon May 8

Wrote two letters one to Dr. Fleming and one R. R. Wallace 74th Ohio. Have not changed camp to day. Forces reviewed by Maj. Gen. Grant – an order read from him complimenting the army on their achievements – amongst the rest gave the number of prisoners captured near Port Gibson at one thousand. Promised the principal part of our hardships would soon be over but said that more battles were first to be fought. Weather pleasant. Warmer than the last two days.

Saturday Eve May 9th 1863.

Weather fine nights rather cool in the after part. Still remain <u>in status quo</u>. Since we left Milliken's Bend have not been sheltered by tents. Arrange a few green boughs to form a shade beneath which we lie lazily during the heat of the day. The same arrangement also suffices to intercept the heavy dews that *fall. Make our beds on the ground and sleep with lizards and snakes with which country abounds.*

Sabbath Eve May 10

Marched nine miles – passed through village of Cayuga – now distant 30 miles from Jackson and 20 from Vicksburg – very disagreeable marching roads extremely dusty. Gen. Sherman with us – our entire force about sixty thousand. Weather sultry. Object perhaps to reach Jackson rather than cross Black River to go to Vicksburg.

NOTES FOR May 10
Jackson, Mississippi: the Mississippi state capital, bordered by the Pearl River to the east. This is about forty-five miles east of Vicksburg.

Tuesday Morning 12th

Did not move yesterday. Reveille at 3 o'clock this morning. Took up line of march at 5 – being near enemy – distant perhaps 10 or 12 miles.

Evening

Marched about 7 miles. Skirmished two or three miles. Two of our cavalrymen wounded don't know what damage the Confederates sustained. Bivouac for the night on the banks of Baker's Creek. Country through which we have passed the last few days very sterile and barren.

NOTES FOR May 12
Baker's Creek: A period map shows Baker's Creek as about twenty-five miles long, lying about two miles east of Edwards Station (Edwards Depot), Mississippi, flowing south into 14 Mile Creek, a tributary of the Big Black River.

Thursday Evening May 14- 1863.

Yesterday morning reveille at day break – moved down on the road towards Edwards Depot within 2 ½ miles skirmishing all the way. About noon we drew off and moved across to the road leading to Raymond – marched during the day about 7 miles and bivouacked in a ploughed field. Heavy rain fell a little before dark made it almost impossible to move – finally changed to a pasture field where we slept fine during the night. Reveille again at daylight this morning. Commenced raining about the time we took up our line of march. Muddy roads raining all day. Still raining with prospect of raining all night. Marched 12 miles to-day. Stopped for the night 4 miles north of Raymond. Raymond a town numbering about 800 – built on a hill. Everything pretty destroyed by the soldiers. Day before yesterday a fight occurred about 2 miles south of town between Gen. Logan's division and the Rebels. Commenced about 10 A.M. and lasted 3 hours – sharp fighting ensued – our loss was from 300 to 500 killed wounded and captured – loss of enemy from 600 to 800. Logan reported about 6 miles south of our bivouac – also Quimby and the whole of McPherson's corps. Sherman's corps reported on our right. Returned to regt this evening Dr. Washburne who was left with our wounded at Port Gibson.

NOTES FOR May 14
Edwards Depot (also called Edwards Station): a small town west of Bolton along the Jackson-Vicksburg rail line.
Raymond: a small town southwest of Clinton, Mississippi. It is about thirty-five miles east southeast of Vicksburg and has a very beautiful court house.

Gen. Logan: (Union) Major General John A. Logan (1826-1886) was a prominent Democratic Illinois congressman whose support Lincoln needed and thus Logan was appointed.

Bolton
Friday, May 15

News rec'd this morning of the capture of Jackson the Capital by Gen. McPherson's corps. Our division moved to Clinton distant 4 miles thence to this station on the Vicksburg & Jackson Rail Road making a march of 12 miles. Arrived here about noon and will probably remain to-night. Clinton on the main rail road route a town numbering about 600 – quite a number citizens there – saw many of the "fair Secesh." We are now between Jackson and Vicksburg distant from the former 15 miles and the latter 40. Campaign so far has been successful beyond my most sanguine expectations. Weather to day cloudy but no rain – roads improving.

NOTES FOR May 15
Bolton: a town west of Clinton along the Vicksburg-Jackson rail line.

Clinton, Mississippi: now a suburb just west of Jackson, in Underhill's time a station along the Vicksburg-Jackson rail line.

Saturday Night May 16- 1863.

Reveille at half past three o'clock this morning. Took up march little after daylight marched westward along a road parallel with the rail road from 5 to 8 miles till we came unexpectedly upon the pickets of the enemy. After reconnoitering as usual we finally made the attack with our division and after a hard fight succeeded in driving the enemy one and an half miles and taking six pieces of Artillery. The enemy however, being largely reenforced numbering three lines our division after a most desperate struggle drove us back over the whole of the ground we had taken but we being reenforced by Quimby's division again drove them back in return and held the field. Our division was under fire 6 ½ hours and lost heavily. Our Regt having perhaps the smallest loss and losing about 75 in killed and wounded. Some are also missing. Quimby's division lost heavily as also did Carr's which were all the troops engaged save a little sparring by General Logan. We are camped to night on the Rebel side of the battle-field. The loss of the enemy in killed and wounded is perhaps fully as great as our own although they had much the advantage in position. Besides their loss in prisoners was very heavy. News received of the capture of Richmond Va: also the occupation of Warrenton.

NOTES FOR May 16
Warrenton: a town in Mississippi on the Mississippi River just south of the mouth of the Big Black River and about eight miles south of Vicksburg.

Sunday Evening May 17th-

Been busy all day and last night in attentions to wounded – wrapped in my blanket and slept one hour last night among the bushes beneath the stars. Entire loss of our division in the battle of yesterday ascertained to be 1,306. Balance of troops save our brigade has gone in pursuit of enemy in direction of Black River. Our brigade remains to bury the dead. Not known when we will follow. Rec'd letters to-day from J. P. Dougal member of 102nd O. V. I. Dr. W. S. Haymond and J. A. McKee also a poem from the latter – weather pleasant.

NOTES FOR May 17
J. P. Dougal: promoted to second lieutenant from first sergeant 1 February 1863; promoted to first lieutenant 8 April 1865.

Tuesday Eve May 19th

Yesterday our division was engaged in burying dead, collecting spoils of battle, etc. This day at noon we took up our line of march and are now on the north bank of Black River, bivouacked for the night – marched 10 miles this afternoon – 15 yet to Vicksburg. Dr. Washburn left with our wounded near the battlefield – country through which we move is barren and desolate –

more level, however, than further down. A sharp fight occurred to our advance at Black River. Since we have landed on this side of Mississippi have taken in all 7,000 prisoners besides their wounded and captured 90 pieces of artillery.

Wednesday Eve May 20.

Remained in camp all day on bank of Big Black River. This evening rec'd orders to go forward towards Vicksburg. Been fighting there to-day and it said we have possession of some of the outer works.

Thursday Evening, May 21.

This evening finds us in camp just back of Vicksburg perhaps 3 miles distant from the city. Last night we commenced our march about dark and marched till midnight when we turned in an old field to rest till morning. I had no blanket so I had an uncomfortable time trying to sleep in the open air with nothing between myself and the ground and no covering of any kind whatever. Latter part of the nights are here at this season of the year decidedly cool no matter how warm may have been the previous day. Took up line of march this morning about sunrise and reached present encampment about 2 o'clock P.M. About noon it rained heavily and most of us were completely soaked. We are now lying in a ravine behind the division of Osterhaus who is in the advance of this corps. Our corps – McClernand's occupies the left – McPherson's the center and Sherman's the right resting on the Yazoo. Haines Bluff has been evacuated. We are plying our Artillery on the enemy and have our sharpshooters so close upon them that they can scarcely get an opportunity to reply.

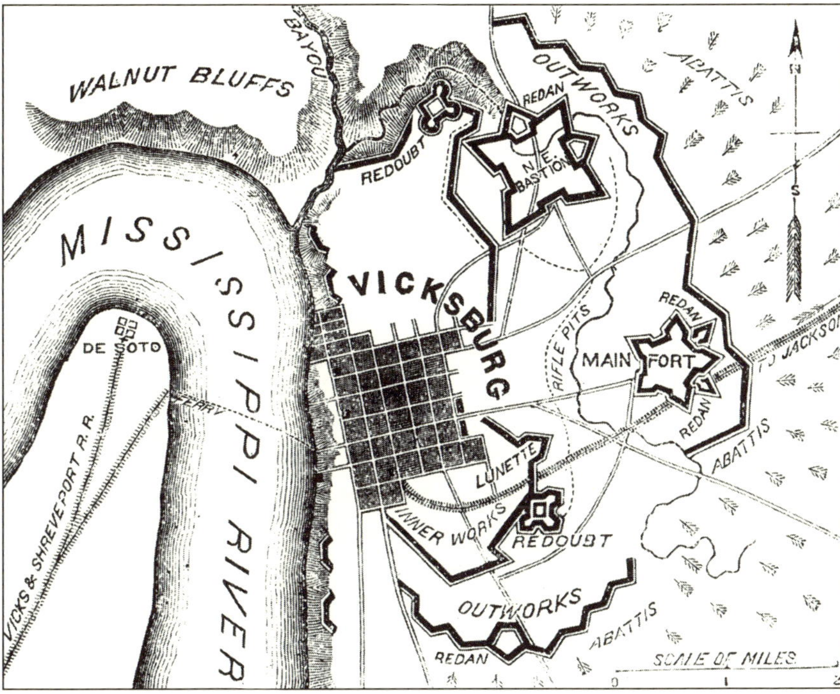

Strongly fortified and surrounded by numerous ravines, Vicksburg held a commanding location on a ridge above a hairpin turn in the Mississippi River. The prominent location of the city made its control a key to controlling the river, and the capture of Vicksburg had long been one of the principal objectives of the Union Army.

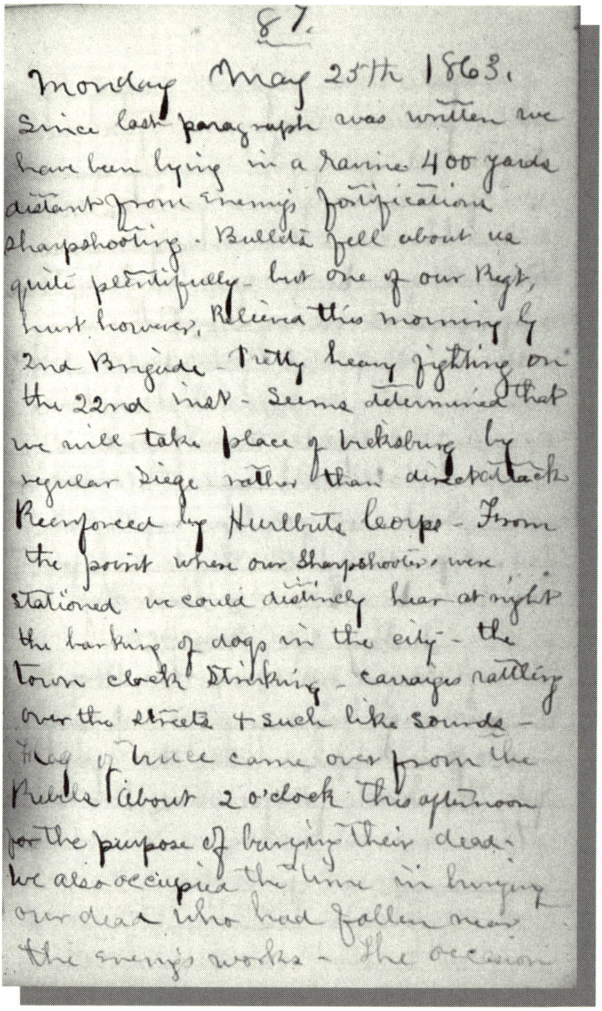

87.

Monday May 25th 1863.
Since last paragraph was written we
have been lying in a ravine 400 yards
distant from enemy's fortifications
sharpshooting - Bullets fell about us
quite plentifully - but one of our Regt,
hurt however, Relieved this morning by
2nd Brigade - Pretty heavy fighting on
the 22nd inst - Seems determined that
we will take place of Vicksburg by
regular siege rather than direct attack
Reenforced by Hurlbuts corps - From
the point where our sharpshooters were
stationed we could distinctly hear at night
the barking of dogs in the city - the
town clock striking - carriages rattling
over the streets & such like sounds -
Flag of truce came over from the
Rebels about 2 o'clock this afternoon
for the purpose of burying their dead.
We also occupied the time in burying
our dead who had fallen near
the enemy's works - The occasion

Monday May 25th 1863.

Since last paragraph was written we have been lying in a ravine 400 yards distant from enemy's fortifications sharpshooting. Bullets fell around us quite plentifully – but one of our reg't hurt, however. Relieved this morning by 2nd Brigade. Pretty heavy fighting on the 22nd inst. Seems determined that we will take place of Vicksburg by regular siege rather than direct attack. Reenforced by Hurlbuts corps. From the point where our sharpshooters were stationed we could distinctly hear at night the barking of dogs in the city – the town clock striking – carriages rattling over the streets and such like sounds. Flag of truce came over from the Rebels about 2 o'clock this afternoon for the purpose of burying their dead. We also occupied the time in burying our dead who had fallen near the enemy's works. The occasion . . .

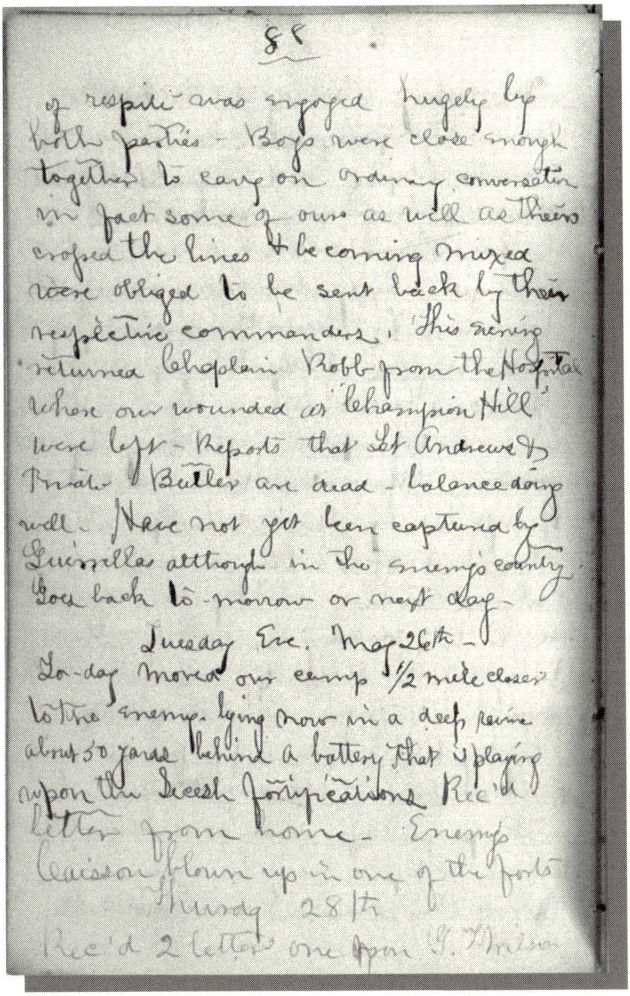
88

of respite was enjoyed hugely by both parties - Boys were close enough together to carry on ordinary conversation in fact some of ours as well as theirs crossed the lines & becoming mixed were obliged to be sent back by their respective commanders. This evening returned Chaplain Robb from the Hospital where our wounded at "Champion Hill" were left - Reports that Lt Andrews & Private Butler are dead - balance doing well - Have not yet been captured by Guirrellas although in the enemy's country. Goes back to-morrow or next day -

Tuesday Eve. May 26th -

To-day moved our camp 1/2 mile closer to the enemy. lying now in a deep ravine about 50 yards behind a battery that is playing upon the Secesh fortifications Rec'd letter from home - Enemy's Caisson blown up in one of the forts

Thursday 28th

Rec'd 2 letters one from [illegible]

. . . of respite was enjoyed hugely by both parties. Boys were close enough together to carry on ordinary conversation. In fact some of ours as well as theirs crossed the lines and becoming mixed were obliged to be sent back by their respective commanders. This evening returned Chaplain Robb from the hospital where our wounded at "Champion Hill" were left. Reports that Lt. Andrews and Private Butler are dead – balance doing well. Have not yet been captured by guirrellas although in the enemy's country. Goes back to-morrow or next day.

Tuesday Eve. May 26th-

To-day moved our camp ½ mile closer to the enemy, lying now in a deep ravine about 50 yards behind a battery that is playing upon the Secesh fortifications. Rec'd letter from home. Enemy's caisson blown up in one of the forts.

NOTES FOR May 25
Gen. Hurlbut: (Union) Major General Stephen Augustus Hurlbut (1815-1882), Commander of the 16th Army Corps of the Army of the Tennessee. He was born in South Carolina but moved in 1845 to Illinois, where he became a prominent Republican and state legislator. He had a bad reputation and was frequently involved in corruption.[32]

Champion Hill: named after the family which owned, and still owns, the property where the battle was fought. The Confederates put up very stiff resistance to keep the Union forces from moving west towards Vicksburg but were finally defeated.

Private William Butler, Co. F, 46th Indiana. Residence: Camden, Indiana. Promoted to corporal. Date of muster: 14 November 1861. Killed at Champion Hill 16 May 1863.

Thursday 28th

Rec'd 2 letters one from G. T. Wilson and one from Linnie. Also 3 papers from latter. Another caisson of the enemy's blown up to-day. Shots fired and aimed by German Deserters. My horse shot and wounded to-day will be crippled perhaps a few weeks.

Friday Eve May 29-

This morning for half an hour from 6 till 6 ½ and this evening from half past 5 o'clock till six a most terrific bombardment took place – without, however, much apparent effect. One house only known to be burned.

Tuesday Eve June 2- 1863.

Regt been on duty last two days as sharpshooters. Last night had three alarms pickets firing occasionally all night – did not get much sleep as a consequence.

Wednesday Eve June 3rd

Wrote two letters one to Dr. W. S. Haymond and one home. This eve the enemy are endeavoring to shell our position – without however, much success. Shots and shell have and are falling all around us but as yet no one of our reg. has been hurt. Regt go on duty to-morrow as sharpshooters.

Friday June 5- 1863.

Still in rear of Vicksburg. Rec'd to-day a letter from Dr. Fleming – yesterday wrote to George T. Wilson. To-day Dr. Coleman went in charge of Ambulance Train to Champion Hill after wounded of our division. Weather very warm.

Saturday June 6-

One year ago to-day we took possession of Memphis. The 43rd and 46th Ind- Regiments constituted all the Infantry. City surrendered after a severe gun-boat fight in which almost the entire Rebel flotilla was destroyed. Today weather warm.

Rear of Vicksburg Miss
Sunday Eve June 7.

To day was killed Andrew J. Bachelor of Co B by the falling in of a bank where a number of soldiers were digging and forming a magazine. He was completely submerged and lived not more than two hours after he was dug out. To-day rec'd and wrote a letter to Linnie.

NOTES FOR June 7
Andrew J. Bachelor: Recruit, Co. B. Residence: Logansport, Indiana. Date of muster 13 February 1862. Died at Vicksburg 7 June 1863 of wounds caused by the collapse of a magazine.

June 8th

To-day Lt George W. Spencer went north having been dismissed the service. A paper – setting forth that he was a zealous patriot and had done everything possible to assist in putting down the Rebellion – was unanimously signed by the officers of the regt. His departure was deeply regretted by all of us. To-day rejoined the regt Quartermaster Downey.

NOTES FOR June 8
Quartermaster Downey: Elza J. Downey. Date of muster: 11 December 1861. Enlisted in Company A and appointed commissary sergeant 11 December 1861. Commissioned quartermaster 12 June 1862. Wounded at Fort Pemberton, Mississippi 4 April 1863 when he was struck in the hand by a Confederate shell. Resigned 15 June 1863.

Rear of Vicksburg – Miss.
Thursday June 11– 1863–

Weather last two days been very rainy. To-day wrote two letters one to Dr. Fleming and one to Jeremiah T. McPherson Bethesda, Belmont Co: Ohio. This is the 23rd day of the siege and still the City has not capitulated. But the end is sure – it may take one week or possibly one month but the end is sure. The fates have decreed it and the city is doomed. Let us hope that the surrender will not be postponed beyond a few days at most.

Sabbath June 14th

Day before yesterday wrote to John Dixon. Yesterday to Annie Lisle – Canton Ohio – Yesterday returned to the reg. Col Bringhurst having been absent a week or two at Court Martial – Milliken's Bend. Quartermaster Downey resigned – Private Jno Shields Co:E discharged – siege still progressing favorably. Yesterday Dr. Washburne rejoined regt. Weather hot during day and cool at night. My bed I make of about 20 cane lashed together over which a blanket is spread and an oil cloth stretched above the whole – forms an easy couch being raised a foot or two above the ground– – –
– – –Prices of a few items – Northern Daily Newspapers 25 cts – Memphis daily 15 – Eggs 50 cts per dozen Butter 75 cts per lb. and other such articles in proportion – California prices –

NOTES FOR June 14.
Annie Lisle: Nothing is known about her.

John S. Shields, Pvt., Co. E. Residence: Monticello, Indiana. Date of muster: 5 November 1861. Discharged 13 June 1863 because of disability. Most likely the son of John, shown in the 1860 census as 49, a farmer from Buffalo in Liberty Township, White County, Indiana, and Catherine, 45. There were six siblings. Shields would have been about 24 at the time of his discharge.

Wednesday Morning June 17

Have been quite unwell the last few days but managed to perform my duties. Am a little better this morning. Siege still progresses favorably. Day before yesterday we discharged J. W. Tippet and Benj. Carmine private of Co B. One year ago today we had the fight at St. Charles on White River Arkansas. Had left Memphis on the 15th.

NOTES FOR June 17
J. W. Tippett, Sgt., Co. B. Residence: New Waverly, Indiana.

Date of muster: 5 November 1861. Discharged 15 June 1863 because of disability.

Benjamin F. Carmine, Pvt., Co. B. Residence: Dover Creek, Indiana. Date of muster: 5 November 1861. Discharged 16 June 1863 because of disability.

Friday June 19- 1863.

To-day rec'd letter from J. P. Dougal. Weather warm. Wounded to-day Solomon Camlin Co G. making 5th wounded here. One killed almost instantly. Gen. McClernand commanding our corps is to be relieved by Major Gen. Ord. Probable cause personal difficulty with Gen. Grant. To be regretted – McClernand is one of our most successful generals second only in military ability to Gen. Grant in this Department and probably not to him. Discharged last two days Thos. Castle, Beneathy and Smith. Siege still progressing favorably. Forty thousand reenforcements at least have at different times been sent here making Grant master of the situation. Herron and Washburne are here also Burnside's corps. Last few days and nights large artillery been throwing hot shot.

NOTES FOR June 19

Solomon M. Camlin, Pvt., Co. G. Residence: White City, Indiana. Date of muster: 5 November 1861. Promoted to corporal. Wounded on the works at Vicksburg, Mississippi. Discharged on account of wounds.

Maj. Gen. Ord: Edward Otho Cresap Ord (1818-1883) was a Union general who relieved Major General McClernand at Vicksburg. He was born in Maryland and graduated from West Point in 1839. He retired in 1881 and died in Cuba of yellow fever in 1883.[33]

Thomas Castle, Cpl., Co. B. Residence: Logansport, Indiana. Date of muster: 5 November 1861. Discharged 16 June 1863 because of disability.

Robert Beneathy, Cpl., Co. D. Residence: Logansport, Indiana. Date of muster: 5 November 1861. Discharged 19 June 1863 because of disability.

Zachariah T. Smith, Pvt., Co. A. Residence: Delphi, Indiana. Date of muster: 1 November 1861. Discharged 19 June 1863 because of disability.

Herron: (Union) Major General Francis J. Herron (1837-1902). A Pittsburgh-born Iowa banker, he was captured at Pea Ridge. He commanded a division in the Army of the Tennessee from 11 June to 28 July 1862, serving in the Vicksburg campaign, later transferring to the Department of the Gulf. At the time he was the youngest major general on either side.[34]

Burnside: (Union) Major General Ambrose Everett Burnside (1824-1881) was born in Indiana and graduated from West Point in 1847. He suffered several reverses on the eastern front, but he was a man of high character who after the war became a governor of Rhode Island and later a senator. He was famous because of his whiskers, known as sideburns.[35]

hot shot: shot heated red hot in order to start fires.

June 20 – 1863.

This A.M. at 4 o'clock all the land artillery nearly 200 pieces in number – the gunboats and mortar fleet opened up on the city – and rained a terrible fire for six hours – Not much visible effect.

Sunday June 21 – 1863.

Wrote letter to-day to J. P. Dougal. Attended divine service in regiment.

Tuesday June 23 –

Rec.d letters yesterday from J. A. McKee, Ross Wallace and Miss L.____J.____. Also two papers from the latter. News rec'd. to-day of the invasion by the Rebels of the State of Pennsylvania.

June 25

This morning at precisely half past 4 o'clock a mine was sprung under a fort opposite to Gen. Logan which he had been undermining for a week or more. Precisely at the time artillery and musketry opened up all around the works to create a diversion. Wrote two letters to day one to Linnie under dates of 23rd and 24th also to Jno. McKee.

June 30 – 1863.

Finished reading a novel "The Hills of the Shatemuc" by the author of the "Wide, Wide World." Tolerably well pleased with the work which may be styled a sort of religious novel. Principal Characters Mr and Mrs. Landholm – two sons Will Rufus, and Winthrop – daughter Winifred – Mr. Haye – Miss Cadwalleder and Miss Lizzie Haye – Mr. Herfed the naturalist and Mr. Underhill. Story ends well. This month have died two members of our reg. from disease – Nicholas Smith Co. B and Wm. T. Davidson Co. C. – last month lost none by disease. Siege progressing favorably. Weather hot and sickness increasing. Sent $200 on 24th inst. to George W. Spencer Monticello, Ind – deposited.

NOTES FOR June 30

The Hills of the Shatemuc (1856) was written by Susan Warner (1819-1885), who lived in Constitution Ward, New York. She also published under the pseudonym Elizabeth Wetherell. Since her name is not given by the publisher, Underhill mentions the book as having been written by the author of *Wide, Wide World*, which was immensely popular in 19th century America. Her works were often of a religious nature. The *Hills of the Shatemuc* appears to be set along the Hudson River. Although names are changed, the use of Mannahatta for a large city suggests New York. Although he does not mention several characters, Underhill has all the names correct except for the naturalist, whose name is Herder. The prose to a modern reader seems stilted and the characters static, and the women seem to cry incessantly. Underhill terms it a religious novel because Mrs. Landholm wants to be sure her sons are true Christians. Winthrop becomes one and eventually influences Elizabeth Haye to become one as well, and at the end he proposes to her.

Nicholas D. Smith, Pvt., Co. B. Residence: Logansport, Indiana. Date of muster: 5 November 1861. Died at Vicksburg 24 June 1863.

William T. Davidson, Pvt., Co. C. Residence: Pittsburg, Indiana. Date of muster: 7 November 1861. Died at Vicksburg 27 June 1863.

Rear of Vicksburg – Miss – July 1 – 1863.

Intelligence has been rec'd that the Rebel Gen. Bragg is reenforcing Johnston at Canton to attack our rear. Two divisions are reported as having already arrived there and the greatest part of Bragg's army following. Yesterday a council of war was held – but the deliberations were of course not made known. A few days will probably bring stirring events. Made up Monthly Report and forwarded to R. B. Jessup Surgeon in Chief of our division. Wrote a letter home.

NOTES FOR July 1

Gen. Bragg: Braxton Bragg (1817-1876). (Confederate) General Bragg was born in North Carolina, graduated in the Class of 1837 at West Point and remained on active duty until 1856, when he left to run his Louisiana plantation. From June 1862 until December 1863 he commanded the western Confederate army. He was not liked by his subordinates.

Johnson: General Joseph Eggleston Johnston (1807-1891) was a Confederate general whom Grant respected. He graduated from West Point in 1829 and later served in the Mexican War. He left the U.S. Army to join the Confederacy in 1861. He quarreled with Jefferson Davis. In 1863 he assumed command of the

Department of the West and in December succeeded Bragg.
Canton: a town in Madison County, Mississippi about twenty-five miles north of Jackson, the capital.

July 2 – Noon –

Day quite warm. Mortars opened out on Vicksburg about midnight and bombarded the place very lively till 6 A.M. to-day. Some pieces of shell falling within our own lines. A fort was mined and blown up yesterday. We captured some prisoners.

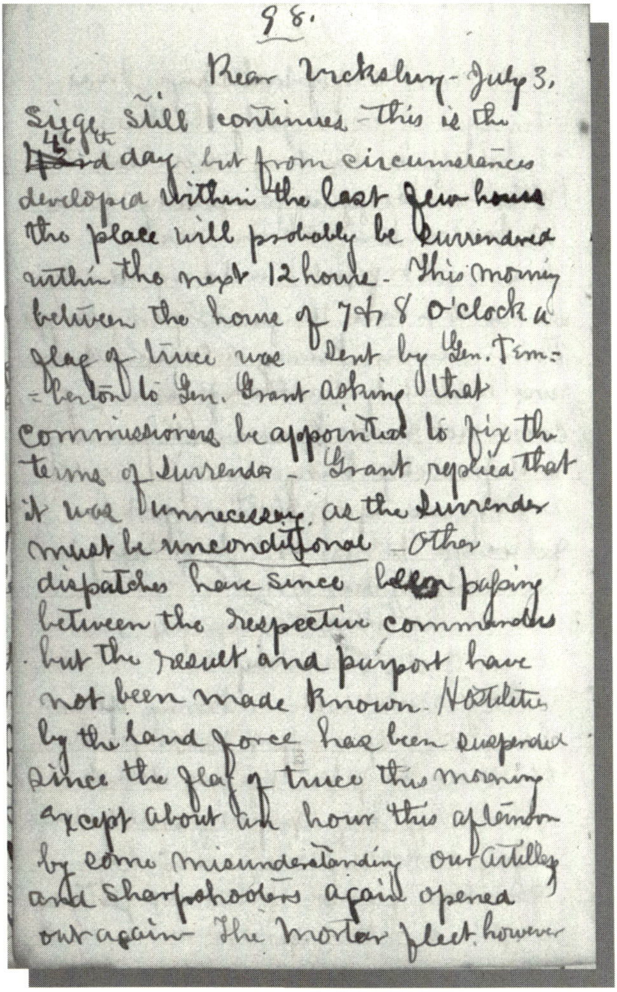

98.

Rear Vicksburg - July 3,

Siege still continues - this is the
46th day but from circumstances
developed within the last few hours
the place will probably be surrendered
within the next 12 hours - This morning
between the hours of 7 & 8 o'clock a
flag of truce was sent by Gen. Pem-
-berton to Gen. Grant asking that
commissioners be appointed to fix the
terms of surrender - Grant replied that
it was unnecessary, as the surrender
must be unconditional - Other
dispatches have since been passing
between the respective commanders
but the result and purport have
not been made known - Hostilities
by the land force has been suspended
since the flag of truce this morning
except about an hour this afternoon
by some misunderstanding our artillery
and sharpshooters again opened
out again - The Mortar fleet however

Rear Vicksburg – July 3.

Siege still continues. This is the 46th day but from circumstances developed within the last few hours the place will probably be surrendered within the next 12 hours. This morning between the hours of 7 and 8 o'clock a flag of truce was sent by Gen. Pemberton to Gen. Grant asking that commissioners be appointed to fix the terms of surrender. Grant replied that it was unnecessary, as the surrender must be <u>*unconditional*</u>*. Other dispatches have since been passing between the respective commanders but the result and purport have not been made known. Hostilities by the land force has been suspended since the flag of truce this morning except about an hour this afternoon by some misunderstanding our artillery and sharpshooters again opened out again. The Mortar fleet, however, . . .*

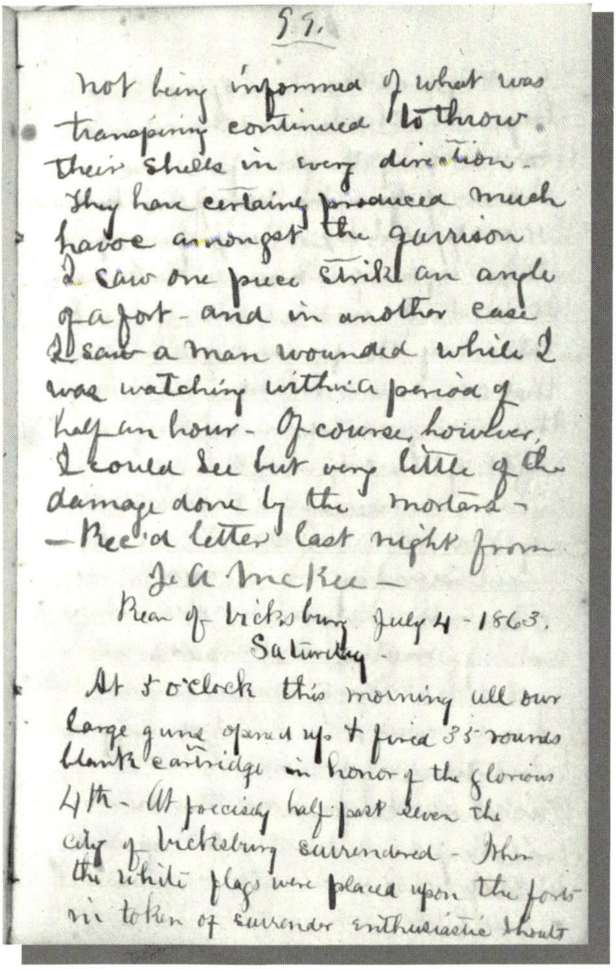
59.

not being informed of what was
transpiring continued to throw
their shells in every direction.
They have certainly produced much
havoc amongst the garrison
I saw one piece strike an angle
of a fort - and in another case
I saw a man wounded while I
was watching within a period of
half an hour - Of course, however,
I could see but very little of the
damage done by the mortars -
- Rec'd letter last night from
J. A. McKee -
Rear of Vicksburg July 4 - 1863.
Saturday -
At 5 o'clock this morning all our
large guns opened up & fired 35 rounds
blank cartridge in honor of the glorious
4th - At precisely half past seven the
city of Vicksburg surrendered - When
the white flags were placed upon the forts
in token of surrender enthusiastic shouts

. . . not being informed of what was transpiring continued to throw their shells in every direction. They have certainly produced much havoc amongst the garrison. I saw one piece strike an angle of a fort – and in another case I saw a man wounded while I was watching within a period of half an hour. Of course, however, I could see but very little of the damage done by the mortars. Rec'd letter last night from J. A. McKee.

Rear of Vicksburg July 4 – 1863.
Saturday

At 5 o'clock this morning all our large guns opened up and fired 35 rounds blank cartridges in honor of the glorious 4th. At precisely half past seven the City of Vicksburg surrendered. When the white flags were placed upon the forts in token of surrender enthusiastic shouts . . .

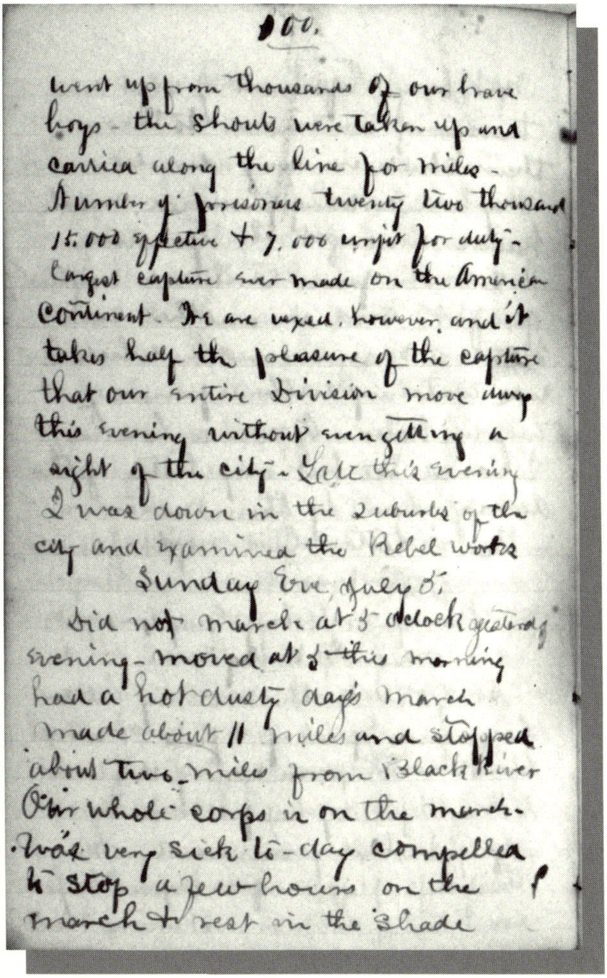
100.
went up from thousands of our brave
boys - the shouts were taken up and
carried along the line for miles -
Number of prisoners twenty two thousand
15.000 effective + 7.000 unfit for duty -
largest capture ever made on the American
Continent. We are vexed, however, and it
takes half the pleasure of the capture
that our entire Division move away
this evening without even getting a
sight of the city - Late this evening
I was down in the suburbs of the
city and examined the Rebel works
Sunday Eve, July 5.
Did not march at 5 o'clock yesterday
evening - moved at 5 this morning
had a hot dusty day's march
made about 11 miles and stopped
about two miles from Black River
Our whole corps is on the march.
Was very sick to-day compelled
to stop a few hours on the
march & rest in the shade

. . . went up from thousands of our brave boys. The shouts were taken up and carried along the line for miles. Number of prisoners twenty two thousand 15,000 effective and 7,000 unfit for duty – largest capture ever made on the American Continent. We are vexed, however, and it takes half the pleasure of the capture that our division move away this evening without even getting a sight of the city. Late this evening I was down in the suburbs of the city and examined the Rebel works.

Sunday Eve, July 5.

Did not march at 5 o'clock yesterday evening – moved at 5 this morning had a hot dusty day's march. Made about 11 miles and stopped about two miles from Black River. Our whole corps is on the march. Was very sick to-day compelled to stop a few hours on the march and rest in the shade. . . . [Heavy cannonading heard this afternoon in a northwesterly direction.]

NOTES FOR July 3
Pemberton: Lieutenant General John C. Pemberton, Confederate general commanding the Army of Mississippi which included the garrison at Vicksburg. Born in Philadelphia, he graduated from West Point in 1837 and served in the Mexican War. He married a Virginian. Jefferson Davis had made him a lieutenant general in order that he outrank generals Van Dorn and Lovell. Many Confederates looked askance at his performance at Vicksburg.

Monday – 10 o'clock P.M.

Been lying under the shade of the oak trees resting all day. March again at 4 o'clock. As the result of fighting heard in the northwest yesterday a large number of prisoners were taken back towards Vicksburg – also an immense number of arms etc. Evidently the campaign is not yet over in the southwest. Day very hot.

Tuesday July 7 –

At 5 o'clock yesterday afternoon got under way and marched 2 miles to Black River Bridge where we camped for the night. Made my bed of two cotton bales.

Wednesday July 8-

Yesterday crossed Black River and marched 16 miles along the Mississippi & Jackson RR to Bolton Depot. Passed over the Battlefield "Champion Hill" which called up many sad memories. The enemy in considerable force under Breckenridge kept ahead of us – occasionally skirmishing a little with his rear. Rained very hard last night and got very wet and could not sleep. No protection from the storm which wet me to the skin making me in a bad humor all day. Of our corps Osterhaus is first in line 2nd Carr – 3rd Smith and 4th Hovey and 5th Lauman – making 5 divisions of the corps – small divisions however. We move again at 5 P.M. to day with 2 days rations and without teams.

NOTES FOR July 8

Breckenridge: John C. Breckinridge (1821-1875) had been Buchanan's vice president and a Democratic candidate for president in 1860. A senator in 1861 from Kentucky, he joined the Confederacy in September, rising to the rank of major general in April 1862. His name appears in various sources both as *Breckenridge and Breckinridge.*

Lauman: (Union) Brevet Major General Jacob Gartner Lauman (1813-1867). Born in Maryland, he was in business in Iowa when war broke out. Attached to Ord's 13th Corps, he was relieved by Ord after disastrous losses in the assault on Jackson, an ouster Sherman and Grant supported.[36]

Clinton – Mississippi
Evening July 9 – 1863.

Did not leave last camp till dark instead of 5 P.M. as expected and also brought all the teams. Marched three miles and lay in the woods till this morning. Started at 7 o'clock feeling our way carefully reached Clinton by 11 A.M. Enemy did not make much of a stand here as expected – skirmished a little – then fell back on Jackson. Clinton is almost deserted not so stirring as when we passed through it in May. Gen. Osterhaus' orderly was taken prisoner by the enemy and shot for having papers permitting him to recruit negroes for the army.

2 miles west of Jackson, Miss.
Friday, July 10 –

Left Clinton this morning – at 8 o'clock arrived here before noon – enemy posted and entrenched in the city and surroundings. Water is difficult of access as all the ponds and cisterns have been rendered unfit for use by the Rebels killing hogs, cattle, mules, etc. and throwing them in the water – a detestable mode of warfare – unfit for civilized nations. Enemy appears pretty formidable. Composed probably of the forces under Johnston reenforced by Bragg. It is known that Breckenridge is there forces number perhaps fifty thousand pretty well entrenched. Ours will number as much besides the cavalry and artillery. Gen. Sherman is in command – Grant having remained at Vicksburg. The different corps of our army have taken several parallel roads till they arrived near Clinton where they converged. Weather hot – will camp to-night in a heavy wood south of the main road.

July 14 – 1863 –

Day before yesterday evening our division moved across to the Raymond and Jackson road passed up that road skirmishing until we struck the Rail Road where we halted and lay on our arms for the night. No one hurt in our brigade. 2 wounded in the 2nd Brigade. Yesterday A.M. about 9 o'clock we again advanced cautiously heavy skirmishing all the time – pushed our division to within 1 ½ miles of the State Capitol our skirmishers having good view of the Rebel works. Our reg't was in the advance lost 8 men wounded – 4 supposed mortally – 11th Ind lost 7 wounded – entire division only about 33. Gen. Lauman's division coming in on our right was more unfortunate. It is said he disobeyed orders and in trying to advance too far was repulsed with severe loss – was immediately relieved of his command which has been temporarily given to our Gen. Hovey. He now commands 5 brigades. To-day we have kept our position gained yesterday which is a very fair one – no one injured to-day in our regiment – several casualties in the other regts. Yesterday two years ago I left home in Ohio which I have not since visited.

1 ½ miles from Jackson on Raymond Road – July 15 – 1863.

This morning finds us still in the same position though it was expected we (our brigade) would have moved across the Rail Road. Our entire corps lay below the Clinton Road – Gen. Osterhaus' division forming the extreme left – next Gen. A.J. Smith's, then Carr's – then on our own and on the extreme right the division which was commanded by Gen'l. Lauman – consisting of 3 brigades. Gen'l. Sherman's corps is next on our left and lastly the 9th Army Corps reaches to the river above town. Thus when our lines are completely closed on the right we will have a line from the river above to the river below. Other troops are arriving. Gen. Lauman's division lost 478 in killed, wounded, and missing on the 13th Inst. News rec'd yesterday of the victory at Gettysburg Penn'a. Dr. Washburn arrived yesterday. Wrote two letters yesterday one home and one to Edgington Ill's – It has been ascertained that the enemy – the soldiers of their army generally – are ignorant of our successes at Port Gibson – Vicksburg and in the East. The principal officers are of course posted as to the truth of the matters. It was determined last night to give to the enemy's pickets our latest papers which will enlighten them.

NOTES FOR July 15

Edgington, Ill's: Edgington, Illinois is in Rock Island County about twenty miles west of Moline. Why Underhill is writing or to whom is unknown, since there are no known family or other connections with Edgington, and no other references to it appear in the diary.

Gettysburg: Scene of fierce battle and President Lincoln's famous address. The Union won two major victories on July 4, 1863: the battle of Gettysburg and the surrender of Vicksburg.

Evening July 16 – 1863.

Yesterday evening the enemy shelled us a little – two passed within a few feet of me while I was eating supper. All night they were very demonstrative – beating drums, sounding calls, etc. An old band of music played "Sweet Home" " Dixie" and "The Bonnie Blue Flag" besides other airs – their music could be heard very distinctly all over our camp – also hear the cars running, locomotives whistling, wagons and artillery rattling over the roads and a thousand other noises. While I write this evening they have again begun to play us some of their Secesh airs on their "brass horns." From the Rail Road I can plainly see the State House and some other large buildings. To-day some heavy fighting to our left – particulars not yet known.

July 17 – Evening

Jackson is evacuated – evacuated last night. Rode over town and fortifications – works were strong enough <u>in themselves</u> but our fire would pass over the first line and annoy the enemy at the opposite side. Might have been flanked. Enemy numbered forty thousand effective men. Town is almost entirely deserted <u>very</u> few families remaining – a desolate place. Boys are pillaging unmercifully – Burning many buildings not only public but private dwellings – Should not be permitted. War, civilized war, is bad enough, it should not be perverted from its original design. Ordered to hold ourselves in readiness to move at a moment's notice – probably return to the Mississippi River in the morning. Rail Road across the Pearl will be destroyed completely. Topography of the country a low plain covered with forest principally dwarf-oak – get water from artificial ponds generally except where we are camped we have access to creek.

NOTES FOR July 17
Pearl River: The river just east of Jackson, Mississippi.

Saturday Evening July 18th

Still bivouacking near Jackson. Ordered to hold ourselves in readiness to move at a moment's warning. Not certain when nor where we will go. Rode down to Pearl River to day. Scarcely as large as Big Black, but a prettier stream not quite so turbid a current and the bed is sandy in some places pebbly – stream rather swift. All bridges over it here have of course been burned by the enemy – fordable, however, near town. Many other buildings burned last night principally store houses and but few private dwellings – done without orders. Saw to-day Harvey Anderson, Jas. M. Swan, Hunt and Stetler old familiar friends from Fairview and vicinity. Enjoyed the visit hugely. They belong to the 30th Ohio Regt. Large detail from our division thoroughly destroying the Rail Road for many miles. Days hot and nights tolerably pleasant. Large numbers of stragglers from the retreating enemy are constantly coming in and being captured – 400 yesterday and 200 to day. Nearly all represent themselves as tired of fighting. A few Rebels have been captured <u>with their paroles in their pockets</u> who were paroled at Vicksburg – will probably be shot for violating their parole. Enemy places torpedoes in the road beyond the river – some have bursted and a few of our men have been killed and wounded – also several citizens killed – a species of guirrella warfare.

NOTES FOR July 18

paroles: How to handle prisoners of war presented challenges to both sides during the war, since maintaining prisoners was a considerable burden. Both informally and later more formally, an arrangement for prisoner exchange was worked out. Essentially, equal numbers of prisoners could be exchanged, although ratios were established whereby one officer was sometimes worth fifteen enlisted men. Prisoners had to go to an official point to be exchanged, Vicksburg being one of these. Once exchanged, they could go back to duty. However, if not officially exchanged, prisoners could be paroled to their own side but were not permitted to undertake military duty until officially exchanged. At Vicksburg after the surrender, Grant had to deal with 30,000 prisoners. Rather than ship them all north and tie up transports hopelessly, he simply agreed to parole them. In this particular instance, parolees, who were forbidden to go back to duty, had done so, with their paroles in their pockets. In essence, they were caught red-handed breaking a rule of the war.

torpedoes: mines

Jackson – Mississippi
Sabbath Evening – July 19 – 1863

Wrote 2 letters one to Jno. A. McKee and one to Lillie Carrelle Canton, Ohio. Rained heavily late last evening. Lt. Fisher and myself slept all night at a house in the suburbs of the city – cloudy and warm to-day.

NOTES FOR July 19
Nothing is known about Lillie Carrelle.

Jackson – Miss. July 20

Rec'd a letter from home also Geo. W. Spencer enclosing note for $200.00. Wrote letter to Fairview – probably move to morrow.

NOTES FOR July 20
There is no evidence showing what the $200 was for.

Raymond, Hinds Co Miss
July 21 – 1863.

Reveille at 2 o'clock this morning – got in line at 3 and moved at 6. Stopped for dinner at Mississippi Springs. Quite a noted watering place. Large buildings to accommodate strangers visiting the springs. Patronized by the soldiers to day. Arrived at Raymond the capital of Hinds Co: this evening –

will bivouac here for the night. Marched 14 miles – country rather barren – road bordered on either side by a pine thicket occasionally a full grown tree.

[Editor's Note:
This is the last entry before Dr. Underhill lost his diary.]

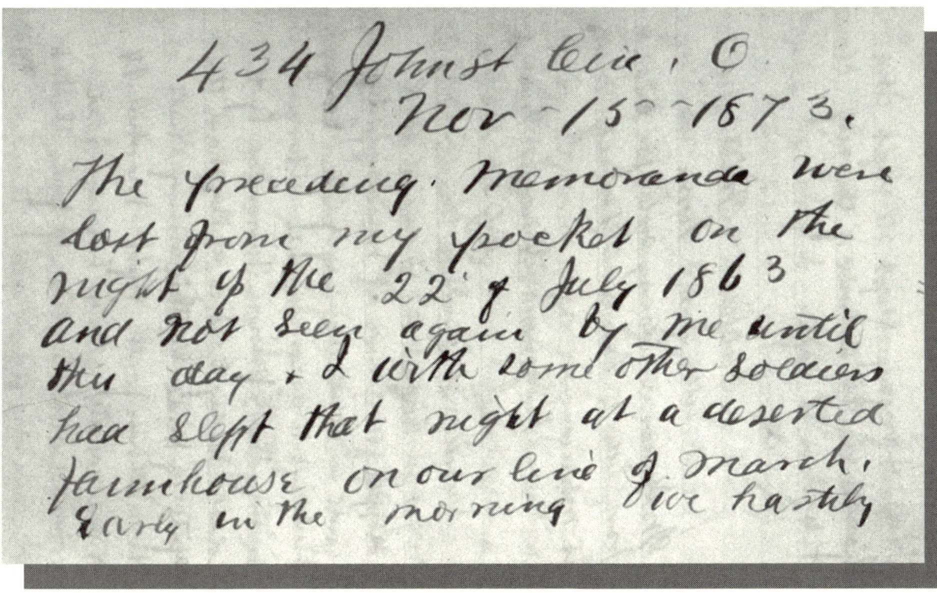

434 John St Cin, O
Nov 15 – 1873.
The preceding memoranda were
lost from my pocket on the
night of the 22 of July 1863
and not seen again by me until
this day. I with some other soldiers
had slept that night at a deserted
farmhouse on our line of march.
Early in the morning we hastily

434 John St. Cin. O
Nov. 15 – 1873

The preceding memoranda were lost from my pocket on the night of the 22 of July 1863 and not seen again by me until this day. I with some other soldiers had slept that night at a deserted farmhouse on our line of march. Early in the morning we hastily . . .

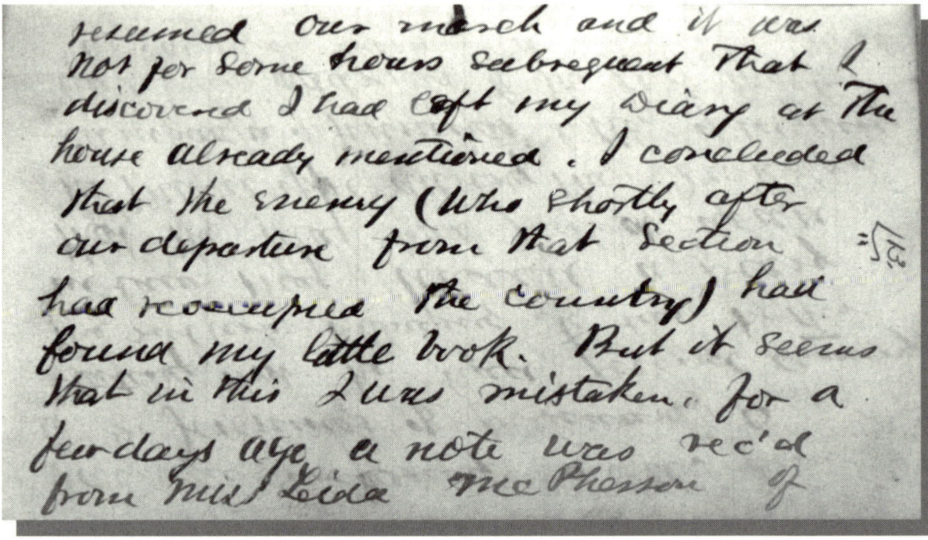

resumed our march and it was
not for some hours subsequent that I
discovered I had left my diary at the
house already mentioned. I concluded
that the enemy (who shortly after
our departure from that section
had reoccupied the country) had
found my little book. But it seems
that in this I was mistaken. For a
few days ago a note was rec'd
from Miss Lida McPherson of

. . . resumed our march and it was not for some hours subsequent that I discovered I had left my diary at the house already mentioned. I concluded that the enemy (who shortly after our departure from that section had reoccupied the country) had found my little book. But it seems that in this I was mistaken, for a few days ago a note was rec'd from Miss Lida McPherson of . . .

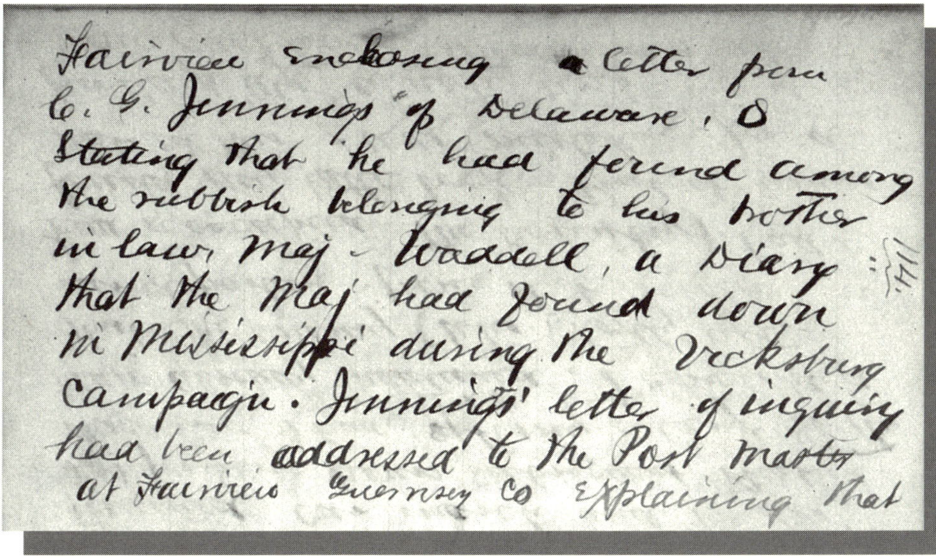
Fairview enclosing a letter fom
C. G. Jennings of Delaware, O
stating that he had found among
the rubbish belonging to his brother
in law, Maj. Waddell, a diary
that the Maj had found down
in Mississippi during the Vicksburg
campaign. Jennings' letter of inquiry
had been addressed to the Post master
at Fairview Guernsey Co Explaining that

. . . Fairview enclosing a letter from C. G. Jennings of Delaware, O stating that he had found among the rubbish belonging to his brother in law, Maj. Waddell, a diary that the Maj. had found down in Mississippi during the Vicksburg campaign. Jennings' letter of inquiry had been addressed to the Post Master at Fairview Guernsey Co explaining that . . .

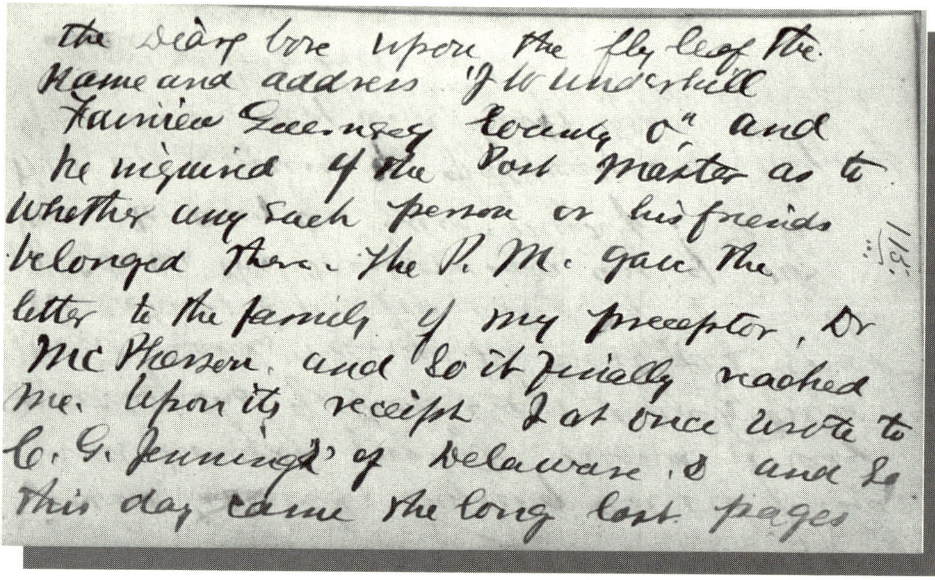
the diary bore upon the fly leaf the
name and address "J W Underhill
Fairview Guernsey County O." and
he inquired of the Post Master as to
whether any such person or his friends
belonged there. The P. M. gave the
letter to the family of my preceptor, Dr
McPherson, and so it finally reached
me. Upon its receipt I at once wrote to
C. G. Jennings of Delaware, O and so
this day came the long lost pages

. . . the diary bore upon the fly leaf the name and address of "J W Underhill Fairview Guernsey County O." and he inquired of the Post Master as to whether any such person or his friends belonged there. The P.M. gave the letter to the family of my preceptor, Dr. McPherson, and so it finally reached me. Upon its receipt I at once wrote to C. G. Jennings of Delaware, O. and so this day came the long lost pages. . . .

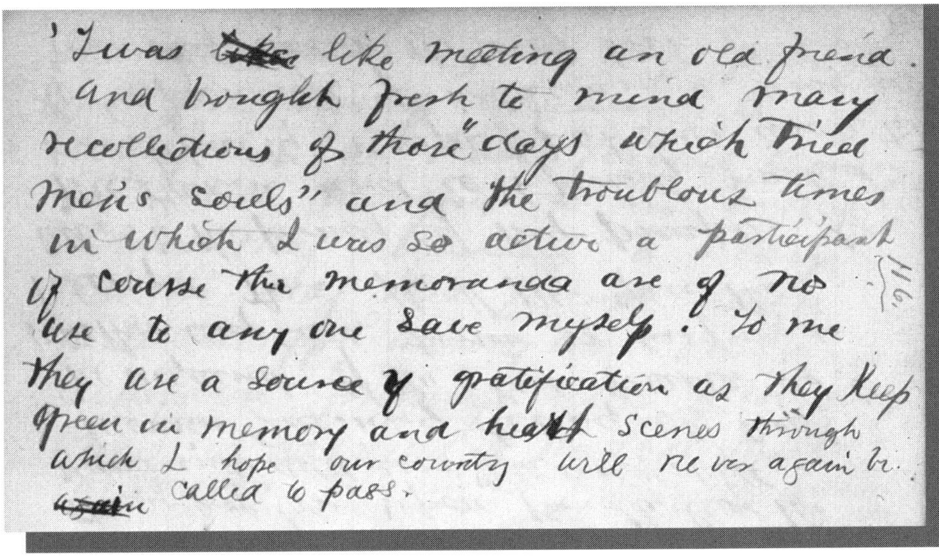

'Twas ~~like~~ like meeting an old friend.
and brought fresh to mind many
recollections of those "days which tried
men's souls" and the troublous times
in which I was so active a participant
Of course the memoranda are of no
use to any one save myself. To me
they are a source of gratification as they keep
green in memory and heart scenes through
which I hope our country will never again be
~~again~~ called to pass.

116

. . . . *'Twas like meeting an old friend and brought fresh to mind many recollections of those "days which tried men's souls" and the troublous times in which I was so active a participant. Of course the memoranda are of no use to any one save myself. To me they are a source of gratification as they keep open in memory and heart scenes through which I hope our country will never again be called to pass. . .*

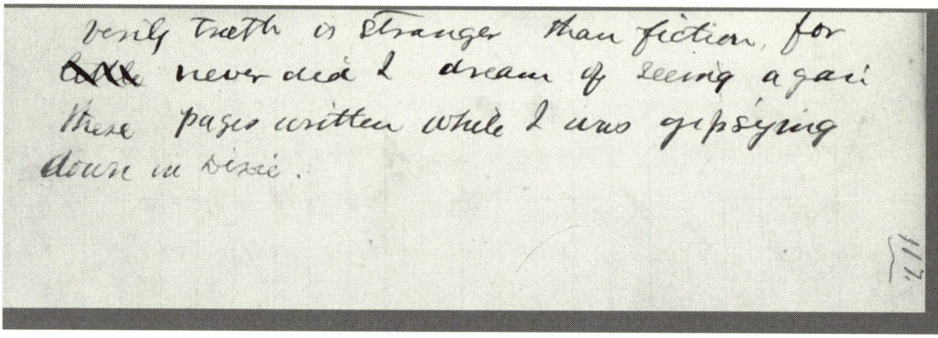
Verily truth is stranger than fiction, for never did I dream of seeing agai these pages written while I was gipsying down in Dixie.

. . . Verily truth is stranger than fiction, for never did I dream of seeing again these pages written while I was gipsying down in Dixie.

NOTES FOR November 15, 1873

Lida McPherson: Eliza McPherson (1849-1894). Daughter of Underhill's medical preceptor Jeremiah T. McPherson and Mary (Gilliland) McPherson, and as of June 16, 1874, Underhill's wife. She is listed on their marriage license as "Lyda," her nickname. In her will she is shown as Eliza McPherson Underhill.

Fairview: Village in Guernsey County, Ohio, where the McPhersons lived prior to moving to Cambridge, Guernsey County, Ohio, in 1876. It was laid out by Mrs. McPherson's grandfather, Hugh Gilliland, Sr., in 1814 and today lies along Interstate 70 about fifteen miles east of Cambridge. Today the village has two main streets but does not appear prosperous. The Fairview Cemetery, on a pretty hilltop south of I-70, is very well kept.

preceptor: When Underhill studied medicine, medical schools were new and often remote. Thus someone wanting to study medicine might instead get his training from a preceptor, a doctor already in practice. Both Dr. McPherson and Underhill's postwar medical partner, Dr. W. H. Dunham, had studied with preceptors.

1889 *1889*

January 15
Bright morning
My Friend were quiet last night comparatively.

NOTES FOR January 15, 1889
This is a cryptic entry. The word *Friend* is not clearly written and it is hard to distinguish the letters. Thus the word might be *friend* or *fiend.* At the time this was written, Underhill was deep in the grip of cocaine addiction and died two weeks later.

End of diary notes:
Henry Snyder: See "Expenses of Mess with Captain Snyder and Lieuts. Spencer & Fisher" at end of diary. Commissioned second lieutenant in Company E of the Indiana 46th, 4 October 1861. Commissioned captain 12 June 1862. Honorably discharged 14 October 1864 because of wounds received at Sabine Cross Roads. Snyder at the end of his life claimed to be the oldest continuous resident in White County, Indiana. He was born in Monticello in 1837 and enlisted in the army immediately upon Lincoln's call, serving for three months before his term expired. He then joined Company E of the Indiana 46th, leaving with the regiment for Logansport the day after his marriage to Charlotte Downs. At the Sabine Crossroads he was wounded when a sharpshooter shot him in the right leg. The ball could not be removed. After being discharged, he returned to Monticello for the rest of his life. His wife died in 1913, and he died in 1918. They had no children.

Graham N. Fitch. See poem entitled "The Mound City" at the end of the diary. First colonel commanding the Indiana 46th, which he raised. Commissioned 20 September 1861. He resigned 5 August 1862. He was born in New York but moved to Logansport in 1843. For several years he held a professorship at Rush Medical College in Chicago. He was elected twice to the Indiana legislature and served four years in the U.S. House of Representatives and four years in the U.S. Senate. In 1860 he supported Breckinridge, who he felt would be able to avert civil war. After the war, Dr. Fitch returned to Logansport.[37]

Editor's Note

The following lists and other material were included in the back pages of the diary and were written before the diary was lost.

Acquaintances in

	Regt.	Co.
Lindsay, J.R.	1st	B
Bumgardner, Henry	"	"
Hinss, C.W.	"	"
Watt, J.W.	"	"
Roseman, William	"	"
Benson, Peter	"	M
Frizzell, R.H.	5	H
Findley, Jos. D.	3rd	A
Cowgill, Frank	15th	B
Penrose, Jno. S.	"	"
Major McClenahan	"	"
Robbins, W.	18th	A
Tillet, Ignatius	25th	A
Belmont County Boys	"	"
McPeek, M.	26	F
Osler, J.	"	"

Ohio Regiments

	Regt.	Co.
Tillet, A.C.	26	F
McPherson, J.L.	27	G
Hays	27	G
Guernsey Boys in	17	
Anderson, T. Harvey	30	I
Miskimmins	"	"
Miskimmins, Allen	4th	H
Acton, Frank	5-21?	A
Wallar, John	62	G
McBride, James	65	H
Stockdales	65	H
Swan, Jas.	"	"
Campbell, Wm. A.	"	"

Acquaintances in

		Regt.	Co.
Dr. William Kennedy	A.S.	64	-
Dillons		"	
Heaney, J.H.		69	B
McCormick, J.D.		74	K
Allison, Omer		"	"
McKee, J.A.		"	"
Wallace, R.		"	"
Findley, R.P. Capt		"	"
Caldwell, Lieut. J.T.	(U.S.S.C.)	76	
McBurney, Wm.		78	H
Giffee, Josiah		85	C
Gleave, David C.		"	"
Two Comps: Guernsey Boys in		97	
Dr. Stewart Asst. Surgeon		97	

Ohio Regiments

	Regt.	Co.
Tuscarawas in	*98*	
Dr. Warfield	*77*	
Pat Dougal	*102*	
Ad Morrow	*120*	
Guernsey Boys in	*115*	
Lt.Col. J. M. Bushfield	*122*	
Guernsey Boys in	*9th*	*Cavly*
Oldham, Thos. Sutler	*122*	
Guernsey boys under Capt. Anderson	*80*	
Guernsey boys in	*122*	*E*
Paxson, Marion	*122*	
Guernsey Boys in	*126*	

Acquaintances in Ohio Regiments

		Regt.	Co.
Paxson, Marion D.		122	
Anderson, Ross	Lieut. 2nd	122	
J. H. S. Correspondent of J. H. Swan			
Guernsey Times- Govingstown, La		30	F
Guernsey Boys 1 Comp		30	F
" "		26	F
Barnesville Boys in		52	
Gleaves (2)		80	
Fuller - (Mrs. Chambers)		80	
Joseph Anderson - Hospital Steward			
40th Reg. Iowa Vol			

Illinois Regiments

	Regt.	Co.
Lieut. Wm. Benton	*9.*	*Cav. A.*
Serg't. Samuel S. Cleland	"	"
John Jamison	*84*	*K*
Ed. Jamison	"	"

Expenses of mess

Date	1862	$	cts
Oct. 10	Tomato Catsup		25
"	Bread		30
" 11	Pepper		10
" "	Eggs		40
" 14	Butter		50
"	Bread		25
" 17	Pork		25
" 20	Bread		50
	Total	2	55
	Settled Oct 31st, 1862		
Nov. 1	Tomatoes (2 cans)	1	00
" 2	Apples & milk		30
" 4	Beef tongue		25
" 10	Cranberries		40
" 23	Cranberries		30
" 26	Fresh Beef		25
Dec. 16	Salaratus		25
Jan. 10, 1863	Beef		25
Jan. 24	Bread		50
Jan. 26	Flour		135

with Capt. Snyder & Lt. Fisher

Date	1863	$	cts
Jan. 31	Beef 12 lbs– 6 ¼ per lb.		75
Feby 3	Beef liver		25
Feby 6	Coffee 2 lbs		68
	Rations Oct. 31st to Dec. 1st	9	00
Feby 12	30 Days Rations	9	00
Feby 25	Coffee 2 lbs		68
"	Bread		25
" 28	Beef	1	00
March	Batch provisions	3	15
2	Beef	1	00
15	Fish		50
20	Batch of provisions	3	60
"	Cheese		25
April	Hospital Boarding	4	50
	Settled up to 1st April	24	63
April	Beef	25	18
May 8th	Coffee & crackers	2	00
"	Bacon & potatoes	2	20
"	Batch of Grub	2	60

Expenses of mess with Capt. Snyder

May 29	*Grub*	*4*	*20*
" 30	*Cod fish*		*40*
June 1st	*Batch of Grub*	*3*	*50*
	Settled up June 2nd –		
Jun 7	*Peaches Dried*	*1*	*10*
8	*Bread*		*50*
Jun 13	*Bread*	*1*	*00*
Jun 14	*Butter*		*50*
" "	*Fish etc.*		*60*
June 19	*Bread*	*1*	*00*
June 21	*Bread*	*1*	*00*
" 24	*Fish*		*30*
" 26	*Tomatoes*		*60*
" 27	*Ginger Snaps etc.*		*50*
" 29	*Grub*	*2*	*65*
" 30	*Honey*		*75*
July 1	*8 lbs. Dried Beef*	*2*	*80*
" 2	*2 loaves Bread*		*20*
" 3	*1 Can Oysters*	*1*	*00*

& Lieuts Spencer & Fisher

July		*$*	*cts*
6th	*Halibut*		*60*
13th	*Bacon & Sugar*	*1*	*50*
	Due Snyder	*1*	*10*
17th	*Settled up to date*		
1863			
July 18	*Provisions*	*3*	*50*
July 20	*Bacon, Rice, etc.*		*90*

[penciled note]

(note 1881
Lieut. Spencer
died a few years
ago a terrible death
from poisoning by
corrosive sublimate
taken by mistake
for quinine

U.)

Landings & Distances
on
White River

Mouth of White River to

Cut Off	*6*
Wild Goose Bayou	*15*
Prairie Landing	*22*
La Gicur	*24*
Ox Bows	*29*
Scrub Grass	*34*
Foot of Little Island	*44*
Head Little Island	*50*
Foot Big Island	*54*
Big Creek	*72*
Indian Bay	*74*
Head Big Island	*78*
St. Charles	*84*
Anderson's Bluff	*85*
Maddox's Bluff	*94*
Crockett's Bluff	*97*
Adam's Bluff	*105*
Cascoe	*115*
Aberdeen	*125*
Rock Roe	*127*
Walnut Ridge	*129*
Clarendon	*135*
Warsaw	*141*

Crooke point Cut off		*150*
Miller's Bluff		*165*
Arkapola		*172*
Duvall's Bluff		*176*
Surrounded Hill		*178*
Lake Bluff		*180*
Hidden Bluff		*185*
Little Hill		*188*
John Wright's		*190*
Wattensour		*192*
Foot Trimble's Island		*193*
Head Trimble's Island		*196*
Capt. Taylor's		*201*
Des Arc		*210*
Arch Hutchins'		*215*
McArtly's		*218*
Pyon's Wood Yard		*222*
Peach Orchard Bluff		*234*
Nigger Hill		*239*
Mouth Little Red		*257*
Gregory's Landing		*263*
Gray's Bend		*273*
Augusta		*282*
Jacksonport	*357*	*357*

Little Red River

from mouth to Searcy's Landing	*45*	*45*

	$	Cts.
Charles Fisher	15	90
Meek	1	30
"		50
Armstrong	1	45
Andrews	5	50
Meek		90
Bishop		50

[Editor's Note: no explanation is given for these figures.]

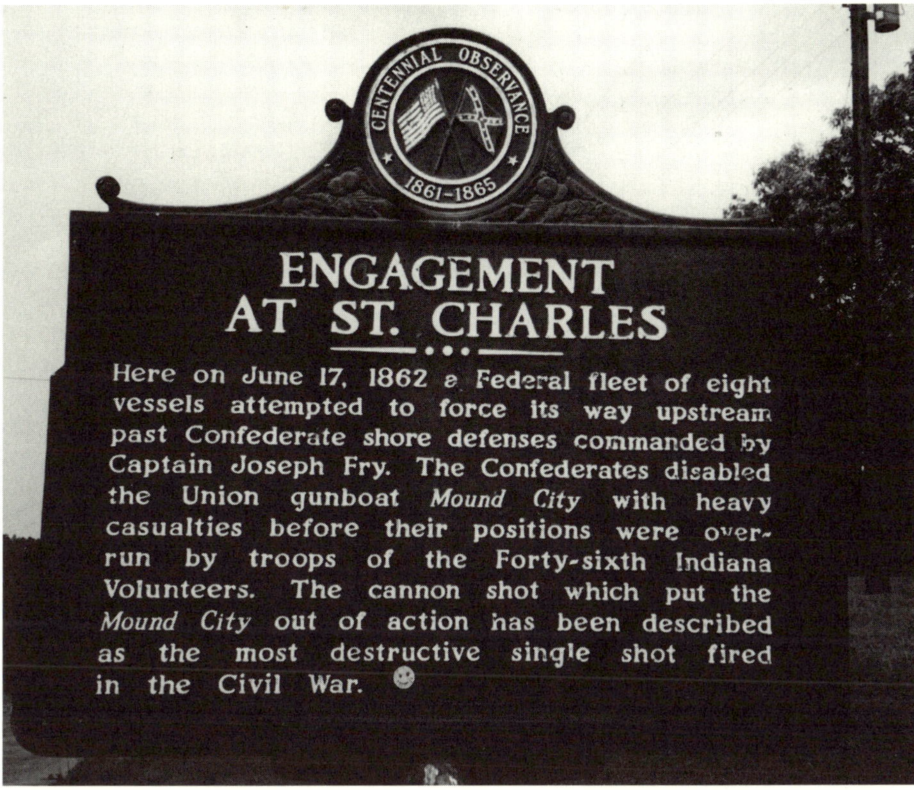

This historical marker erected by the Arkansas Civil War Centennial Commission in 1964 commemorates the fight at St. Charles, Arkansas. The White River lies in the background, at the left. A monument in the center of the town pays homage both to Confederate and Union troops.

[The following lines were written for a New York illustrated paper on the fight at St. Charles, White River, Ark's. on June 17, 1862. The 46th Ind. was only Infantry engaged – the gunboats were the "Cincinnati," "Carondelet," "Lexington," and the ill-fated "Mound City." A 64 pound shot, penetrating the Mound City," cut the connecting pipe, whereupon every portion of the boat was filled with hot steam, scalding to death the entire crew of about 175 – except some 25 who were slightly burned.]

The Mound City
by Charles D. Gardette

Now, gallant Kelly, hold your hand,*
You've done enough to-day.
And give my Indiana braves
A chance to show these lords of slaves
Ten minutes' bayonet play.

Thus through the hissing shot and shell
Stout Fitch's+ signal flew;
The swarthy gunners ceased their toil
and, reeking with the battle moil,
Mute stood the panting crew.

There was a moment's wild suspense,
While many a straining glance
From eyes bloodshot with combat burned,
In rays of focal fire, full turned
Upon our troops advance.

One moment strangely still they stood;
Then, through the lambent air,
As if a thousand fiends astride
Of every sulphurous cloud did ride,
In shrieking triumph there,

A winged demon ball swooped down
Rending the battle gloom,
As through the rifts of thunderous sky,
Rent by Heaven's dread artillery,
Flames down the bolt of doom.

It struck. There was one hideous crash,
One long demoniac scream –
Oh, God! The nightmare of a life
Red with the massacre of strife,
To this were one soft dream!

Oh, sight to wring hot tears of blood
From eyes all strange to tears;
Oh, Sounds to bid dead pulses leap,
And, in a single heart-pang, heap
The agony of years!

A hundred dauntless men, and more,
Stood there in pride but now;
A hundred souls in Heaven they claim,
With "hero-martyr" writ in flame
On each translucent brow!

* * * * *

There is another strain to sing,
Divinely soft and low
Of hearths all ashen, cold and lone
Of homes, through whose dim hall a moan
Like the sad night-wind doth go.
Alas for these, and thrice alas!
Yet shall they kiss the rod:
There is a joy beyond the grave
For those – their hallowed dead – who gave
Their Lives to Freedom's God!

* * * * *

**The "Gallant Kelly" here mentioned was the Captain of the Mound City.*
+*Fitch – The Col. Com'md'g 46th Indiana*

J. W. Underhill
Ass't. Surgeon 46th Ind. Vol. Inf.
Helena, Arkansas
February 6, 1863

End Notes to the Diary and Notes

1 Frederick Way, Jr., comp., *Way's Packet Directory, 1848-1994* (Athens: Ohio University Press, 1994) 289.

2 Stewart Sifakis, *Who Was Who in the Civil War* (New York: Facts on File, Inc., 1988) 320.

3 Sifakis 693-694.

4 Way 155.

5 Way 188.

6 Sifakis 256-257.

7 Sifakis 101-102.

8 Way 437-438.

9 Way 55-56.

10 Way 400.

11 Sifakis 51.

12 Way 179.

13 Sifakis 556.

14 Way 71.

15 Sifakis 95.

16 Sifakis 526,527.

17 Sifakis 650.

18 DeWitt C. Goodrich and Charles R. Tuttle, *An Illustrated History of the State of Indiana* (Indianapolis: Richard S. Peake & Co., Publisher, 1875) 676.

19 Way 473.

20 Sifakis 415.

21 Sifakis 315-316.

22 Sifakis 600.

23 Way 151.

24 Way 327.

25 Way 23.

26 Way 237.

27 Way 455.

28 Way 211.

29 Way 169.

30 Sifakis 424-425.

31 Sifakis 660.

32 Sifakis 329.

33 Sifakis 478-479.

34 Sifakis 305.

35 Sifakis 93.

36 Sifakis 375.

37 Goodrich and Tuttle 633-634.

BACKDROP

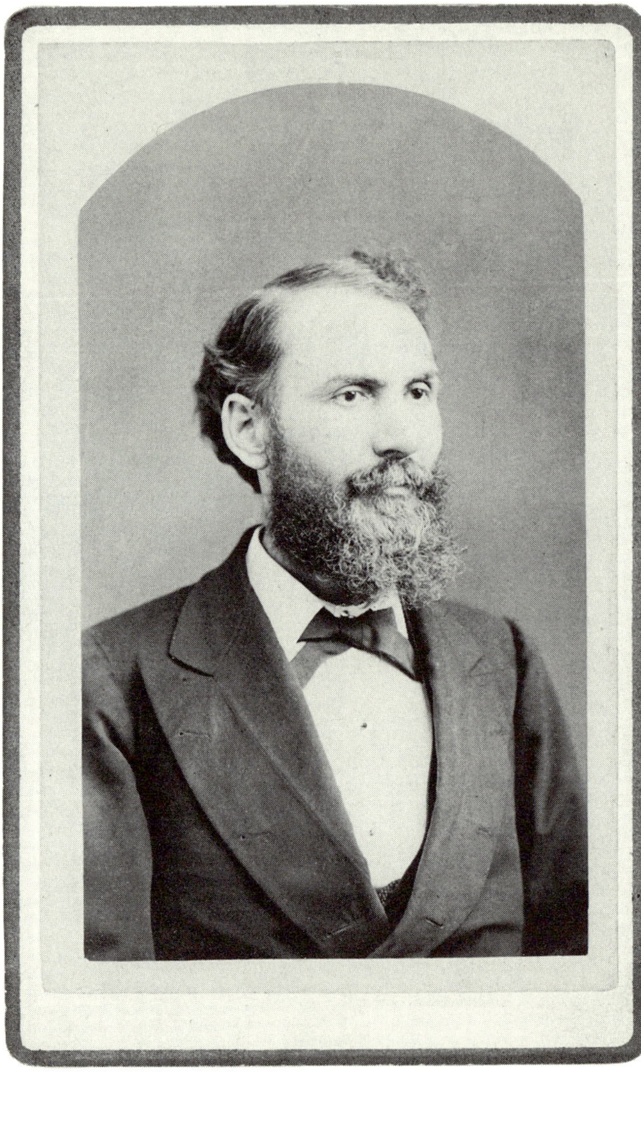

Joshua Whittington Underhill was living in Cincinnati, Ohio, when this picture was taken of him around 1883. Although he was born in Maryland and served with the 46th Indiana Volunteer Infantry during the Civil War, he spent most of his life in Ohio, dying in Cincinnati on 28 January 1889.

Origins

Joshua Whittington Underhill was born January 11, 1837, in the waning days of Andrew Jackson's administration, in Quindocqua, Somerset County, Maryland, on the Eastern Shore close to the Virginia border. Quindocqua, then a settlement of several hundred, is about nine miles from Princess Anne and five miles from Crisfield. Joshua's parents were Thomas Henry Underhill and Eleanor Connor (Whittington) Underhill, who had been married in June 1835 in Somerset County. They had one more child, name and gender unknown, who died in infancy in Ohio about 1840.

The genealogy of much of Thomas Henry Underhill's family has not been positively established, but it is believed that those Underhills who settled in northern Virginia and Maryland came from a separate branch of the family and were not descended from Captain John Underhill who accompanied John Winthrop in the settlement of Boston nor from another Captain John Underhill who settled in Virginia in 1651.

According to the Underhill genealogy,

> The earliest reference to an Underhill actually living in an Eastern Shore county is dated 1728, when an inventory was filed on the estate of Thomas Underhill. Nothing more is known about him, but the date, the fact that he definitely lived on the Eastern Shore, and the popularity of the name Thomas in the later generations of the family all point towards his being the family

> founder. Subject to further research, he has tentatively been given that position.[1]

If this information is correct, this Thomas Underhill was the great-great-great grandfather of Joshua Whittington Underhill.

The grandfather of Joshua Whittington Underhill, also a Thomas Underhill, was born in the 1770s, probably in Virginia, and is thought to have died in the 1840s in Somerset County, Maryland, since he does not appear in the 1850 census. On January 30, 1799, he married Leah Powell, whose mother is unknown, but whose father, Jesse Powell, was born in Somerset County, Maryland about 1743 and died there about 1811.

Thomas and Leah (Powell) Underhill had three daughters: Betsy, Polly, and Rachel, Rachel being the aunt whom Underhill mentions in his diary. Born about 1810, she married John C. Johnson in September 1831 and lived at Snow Hill, Worcester County, Maryland, dying there August 3, 1887. Polly was born about 1808. Betsy, born about 1806, married Thomas Jones on March 12, 1828. She later married someone named Lee and died in Baltimore in 1883.

Thomas and Leah (Powell) Underhill also had three sons: George, born probably about 1820; William J., born in 1816; and Thomas Henry, born in 1814, the father of Joshua Whittington Underhill. The 1820 Somerset County census shows two males under age ten in the household of Thomas Underhill, and since William J. and Thomas Henry lived into adulthood, it may be that George was born after that census was taken.

Joshua Whittington Underhill's mother, Eleanor Connor Whittington, also shown as Nelly Connor Whittington, was the daughter of Thomas and Sarah S. (Connor) Whittington and was descended from Captain William Whittington of the Virginia Militia, who had come from England and settled in Northampton County, Virginia. Thomas was a slave owner, and in his will dated 28 May 1818, he left "unto my loving wife Sarah Whittington all my estate real and personal, all at her dis-

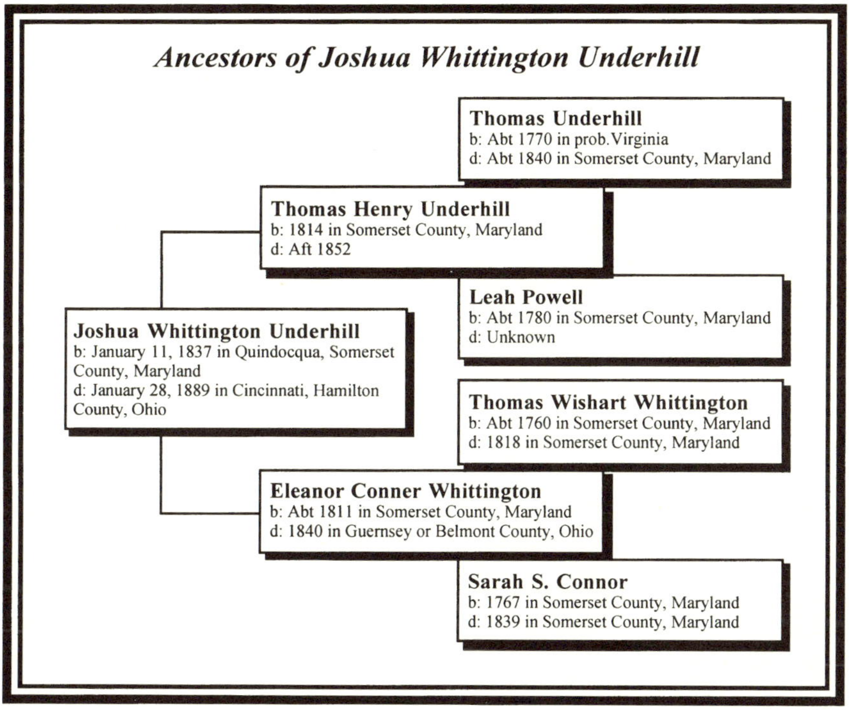

posal except one Negro boy Henry I give unto my daughter Nelly Connor Whittington...."

Eleanor, or Nelly, was born probably about 1810 or 1811. The youngest of seven children in the family, she had five brothers and one sister. Her brother Joshua is thought to have died young or moved west, and it is wholly possible that Joshua Whittington Underhill was named for his uncle. Her sister, Elizabeth (Betsy), was born in 1797 and married William Wilson on January 17, 1817. Their son, George T. Wilson (1819-1889), who lived near Quindocqua on his family's farm in Burnettsville, Maryland, was Underhill's first cousin and is mentioned in the diary.

Although not much is known about Joshua Whittington Underhill's early life, what is known comes from several sources. The Underhill genealogy provides firsthand information dated 1886 from Joshua Whittington Underhill's first cousin. He reported that Joshua's father, Thomas Henry Underhill, had left Somerset County before 1845 and had not been heard from in many years.[2]

Another account appears in a biographical sketch by Otto Juettner, who wrote that Joshua Underhill "was raised by a childless couple, his mother having died when he was three years old, and his father having left for parts unknown and never being heard from any more."[3]

Additional information comes in a short biography by Arthur G. King, which appears in his centennial history of the Cincinnati Obstetrical and Gynecological Society, of which Underhill was a founder. King used Juettner as one source but went on to explain that Thomas and Eleanor Underhill were en route from Maryland to Missouri when they stopped in Belmont County, Ohio, which borders what is now West Virginia. There Eleanor died of childbed fever and the newborn baby from lack of nourishment.[4]

Another account of Joshua Whittington Underhill's youth appeared in *The Cincinnati Enquirer* the day after his death in Cincinnati on January 28, 1889. The newspaper reported that his mother had died in 1856 and that his father, a sea captain, then shipped for South America and was never heard from again.[5] When Joshua Underhill died, his estranged wife, Eliza (McPherson) Underhill, was living in Cambridge, Ohio, and she did not arrive in Cincinnati until the day after the first news article about him appeared. Her sister's husband and later Underhill's administrator, Dr. William H. Dunham, had known him well for many years, and it was he who made the funeral arrangements, but even Dunham was unable to supply Underhill's mother's name, since it does not appear either on the record at Spring Grove Cemetery in Cincinnati or in the newspaper. Where the newspaper got its information is unknown. It is unlikely that anyone in Underhill's family was consulted, and part of the report about him appears erroneous.

When Eleanor (Whittington) Underhill died, Thomas Henry Underhill found himself a widower in his mid-twenties, far from home, and responsible for a three-year-old son. How it came to pass is unknown, but as Juettner reported, Joshua was left in the care of a childless couple. Thomas left, and all the accounts concur that he was never heard from again.

Although Thomas Henry Underhill was not heard from again, strong evidence suggests that *The Cincinnati Enquirer's* report that he had shipped for South America is wrong. The Underhill genealogy cites the 1850 census to place him in Perry Township, Brown County, Ohio, a carpenter with a second wife, Catherine, 27, born in Pennsylvania, and three daughters by her: Mary E., age 7; Henrietta, age 4; and Eunice A., age 2.[6] The evidence that this Thomas Underhill is Joshua Whittington Underhill's father is compelling. He is listed as Thomas H. Underhill, born in Maryland, and age thirty-six, which would be correct, given Thomas Henry Underhill's birth date of 1814.

Brown County, Ohio vital records show that Thomas H. Underhill married Katherine Crosson – shown both as Catherine and Katherine in Brown County records – on September 11, 1842, probably at St. Martin's Church, near Fayetteville, Perry Township, Ohio. Father William Cheymol, a native of Bas Auvergne, Clermont, France, who had been appointed in 1839, conducted the Roman Catholic ceremony. Thomas was about twenty-eight and Katherine about nineteen.

Thomas was Protestant, but in the church cemetery at nearby St. Patrick Fayetteville, a Catholic church founded in 1837, is a marker for Mary Crosson, very likely Katherine's mother, who emigrated from County Donegal, Ireland in 1815 and died February 14, 1847, at age fifty-one. St. Martin's had been founded in 1830 and Mary Crosson was one of the earliest members of the congregation. Why she was not buried at St. Martin's cannot be accounted for, but the one hint besides her name and age that she was probably Katherine's mother is that Thomas and Katherine's oldest daughter was also named Mary.

In addition to the record of Thomas' marriage, there are several deeds recording land transactions by Thomas and Katherine, the earliest the sale of a parcel in Fayetteville, Perry Township, in August 1844, and the latest the sale of another parcel in Fayetteville February 26, 1852. Thus it can be said with certainty that Thomas was alive at that date.

After early 1852, Thomas cannot be traced. Neither Thomas nor Katherine appears in the 1860 census of Brown County, although, interestingly, the 1860 Cincinnati census lists a Catherine Underhill, age thirty-eight and born in Pennsylvania, living as a servant in the house of Jacob Fell, a tanner. She is listed by herself, with neither children nor husband. Her age and place of birth, and her somewhat uncommon last name, coincide with the Katherine married to Thomas H. Underhill in Brown County, Ohio, in the 1850 census. If so, she may by then have been a widow, but there is no accounting for their daughters, Mary, Henrietta, and Eunice, who by 1860 should have been around seventeen, fourteen, and twelve.

What eventually happened to Thomas Henry Underhill and his second family remains uncertain. It is altogether likely that Joshua never knew about his father's second family. No evidence exists that he ever went in search of his father. He mentions neither parent in his diary, and his daughters Nelle and Eliza never mentioned Thomas Henry Underhill or Katherine or children of a second marriage, who would have been aunts.

Also uncertain is whether Thomas abandoned Joshua or simply left him, intending one day to come back to reclaim him. Brown County lies in southwest Ohio, about thirty-five miles east of Cincinnati, far from Guernsey and Belmont counties where Joshua was reared. Given communications in that day, Thomas could easily have disappeared if he wished. Although it is possible that he was illiterate, he seems not to have wanted to stay in touch either with his son or with his family in Maryland.

When his father left, Joshua was taken in by John and Eleanor Gilbert, who at that time were living in Hendrysburg, Ohio. Eleanor, whose name appears as Elenor on her gravestone but who was called Nelly, was born about 1797 and her husband about 1803. The 1840 census shows John Gilbert in Belmont County, Ohio, the residents in his household being one male age 30-40, one female age 40-50, and one male under 5. The census is dated October 24, 1840, which suggests that Joshua was living with them by that time. Neither of his parents appears in that census, and given Juettner's claim that Joshua was three when his mother died, it seems reasonable to assume that Eleanor was dead by that time. While her exact date of death is unknown, it must have been between January 11, 1840, when Joshua would have turned three, and before the October 24 census date. In light of this, *The Cincinnati Enquirer's* report that she died in 1856 appears incorrect, since Joshua would have been nineteen at the time.

Although Joshua may have been little older than three and a half when he moved to Ohio, he seems to have had an early threshold of memory. In a diary entry of March 26, 1863, he notes having received a letter from "George T. Wilson resident of Burnettsville Somerset County Maryland – represents my friend Elijah Ward as going Secesh." Ward, four months older than Underhill, had been a neighbor in Quindocqua, and Underhill must have had a vivid memory if he were to have remembered both Ward, a playmate, and Wilson, a considerably older first cousin who lived in an adjoining settlement. While no evidence exists, it is conceivable, however, that Underhill may have returned to Quindocqua as a young man to visit with relatives and thus had more recent memories than those of early childhood.

Sometime between 1840 and 1850, the Gilberts, along with young Joshua, moved from Hendrysburg to nearby Fairview, Guernsey County, Ohio. Guernsey County adjoins Belmont County on the west, and Fairview sits on the county border. A village with an 1850 population of 444, it had two main streets, laid out in 1814 by Hugh Gilliland, Sr., along the old Wheeling Road, in hilly country about thirty miles west of Wheeling. In the modern day, Interstate 70, the main highway between Wheeling and Columbus, cuts straight through Fairview, leaving intact the two original streets but otherwise cutting in half a village that does not appear prosperous. In both the 1850 and 1860 censuses, Joshua Underhill is shown by name in Fairview, Oxford Township,

Guernsey County, Ohio, living with the Gilberts at ages thirteen and twenty-three, respectively, and in 1860 listed also as a doctor.

Fairview was farming country, and in his youth Joshua Underhill worked on farms. However, he was bright, had academic drive and self-discipline, and apparently without formal schooling, learned to read and write. As a late teenager, he taught school for a couple of years until he earned enough money for the first two years of college, in Antrim, Ohio, in northeast Guernsey County. The Rev. Samuel Findley had started a small preparatory and higher learning institution there in 1835 which officially became Madison College in 1839. By 1842, Madison was coeducational, and it is quite possible that several women referred to in the diary were friends from college days. The curriculum was largely classical, since many students were headed for the ministry, and Underhill would have had Latin and Greek as well as Roman and Greek history and several mathematics courses. The college closed at the outbreak of the Civil War, after a large and controversial building had been constructed which could not be paid for.

Underhill probably attended Madison in the 1856-57 and 1857-58 years. Underhill speaks in several diary entries of his college friend, John A. McKee. Muskingum College records show that a J. A. McKee from Cambridge, Ohio attended in 1857-58, in the Scientific Department of the Muskingum Preparatory Department. Assuming this to be the same McKee, Underhill may have known him in 1856-57. Underhill also speaks of his friend from Richland County, Ad Morrow, whose acquaintance he made in 1857-58. While Underhill does not mention Morrow as a college friend, it seems highly possible that they met at Madison.

After two years of college, Underhill began to study medicine. In that era, when medical schools were in their infancy and often remote, many doctors got their training with a preceptor, a doctor already in practice. This Underhill did, most likely in 1858-59 and 1859-60, with Dr. J. T. McPherson, who was living with his wife and their three daughters in

Fairview. Underhill would eventually marry their oldest daughter, Eliza, in 1874.

Jeremiah Townsend McPherson was twelve years older than Underhill, having been born near Fairview August 22, 1824. After his parents died when he was very small, his uncle and aunt, John and Eleanor (McPherson) Gilbert, then living near Hendrysburg, Ohio, in Belmont County about five miles east of Fairview, brought him up. These are the same Gilberts who later took in Underhill, which explains how Underhill knew McPherson.

McPherson was educated in the local school and then studied medicine with Dr. James W. Warfield (1811-1871), who in 1840 was living with his wife, Rebecca, and numerous children in Fairview. McPherson did take a special course at the Starling Medical College, later to become the Ohio State University College of Medicine at Columbus, but when he did this cannot be positively established. One obituary implies he took this immediately following his training with Dr. Warfield, while another gives the date as 1876. The latter appears more likely, since the college was founded in 1848, by which time McPherson must already have been in practice. The college records do not list Jeremiah Townsend McPherson, although both a handwritten source there and the 1874-75 catalog list a J. M. Townsend as a student but not as a graduate. Whether McPherson's names were reversed or whether J. M. Townsend was a different person, we cannot know.

McPherson practiced in Fairview until 1876, when he moved to Cambridge, Ohio, a considerably larger town about fifteen miles west and the seat of Guernsey County. There he eventually built an imposing two-story stone house on Wheeling Avenue, at the southwest corner of Sixth Street, just up the hill from the railroad station, and as of the mid 1990s, the site of the Guernsey Bank.

While not much is known about McPherson's genealogy, considerably more is known about his wife's ancestry. On April 25, 1848, McPherson married Mary Wilson Gilliland, born in Belmont County, Ohio, the daughter of Nancy (Kennon) Gilliland and Hugh Gilliland, Jr. The senior Hugh Gilliland had moved his family from Virginia to the area about 1806, having sent ahead several of his sons to prepare for the rest of the family to arrive, and in 1814, he was to lay out the plan for the town of Fairview.

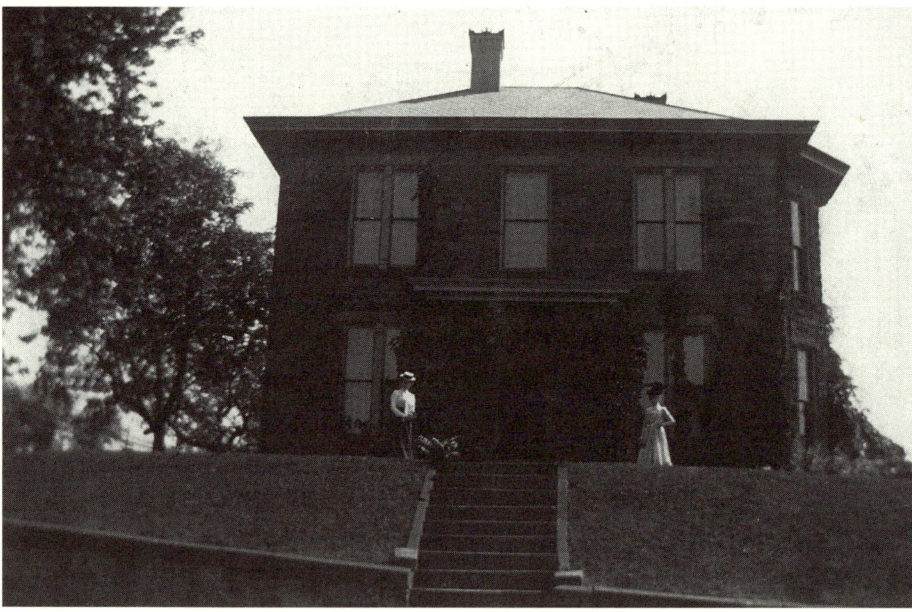

Underhill's in-laws, Dr. Jeremiah Townsend McPherson and Mary (Gilliland) McPherson, move into a new house about 1880 which they built on Wheeling Avenue in Cambridge, Ohio. It was the first stone residence in Cambridge, and the McPhersons lived here for the rest of their lives. In 1894 the house was deeded to Underhill's widow, Eliza (McPherson) Underhill, who had also lived here for some years. Her children later deeded the house to their uncle, John M. Ogier, who sold it to S.W. Nicholson. In 1916, the Cambridge Loyal Order of Moose acquired the property, eventually tearing down the house for a new Moose Hall. A bank now stands on the site of the McPherson house, seen in a photograph taken about 1890.

Nancy (Kennon) Gilliland's father, John Kennon, of Scottish descent but born in County Down, Ireland, had come to America about 1792. In 1794, John married Elizabeth Withney, born in Pennsylvania, and the daughter of a Revolutionary War soldier. They arrived in Guernsey County about 1806, after moving over from Uniontown, Fayette County, Pennsylvania, where six of their ten children had been born, including Nancy in 1795.

Life on the frontier in Ohio was hard. According to a county history published in 1943, the family's first quarters consisted of a primitive hut with bark siding and brush on poles for a roof, until a log cabin twelve feet square was built.[7] Elizabeth (Withney) Kennon insisted on schooling her children despite the rigors of the frontier, and after a few more families moved in, a small schoolhouse was built, where she became the teacher.

Several of her children went on to become highly distinguished citizens. John Kennon, Jr., became a noted surveyor; Newell Kennon held a Treasury Department post in Washington, D.C. and was later a probate judge; William Kennon was a lawyer and judge in St. Clairsville who also served in the U.S. Congress in the 1830s, later becoming a justice of the Ohio State Supreme Court; and Henry Kennon eventually moved to Princeton, Illinois where he too became a judge. On June 16, 1818, their sister Nancy Kennon married Hugh Gilliland, Jr.

Although their daughter Mary (Gilliland) McPherson's date of birth is not known, it was about 1823, for when she died in 1893, her obituary listed her age at about seventy years, the same notation appearing in the family Bible. She loved raising animals, and even after the McPhersons moved to Cambridge in 1876, they still kept a farm a mile or so west of the town, where they raised fine Devon cattle. When Underhill first knew the McPhersons in Fairview, they had three young daughters: Eliza, born in 1849 and named for Mrs. McPherson's sister; Mary, born in 1850 and named for her mother; and Jennie, born in 1857.

After studying medicine with Dr. McPherson, Underhill then completed

Children of Jeremiah T. and Mary (Gilliland) McPherson

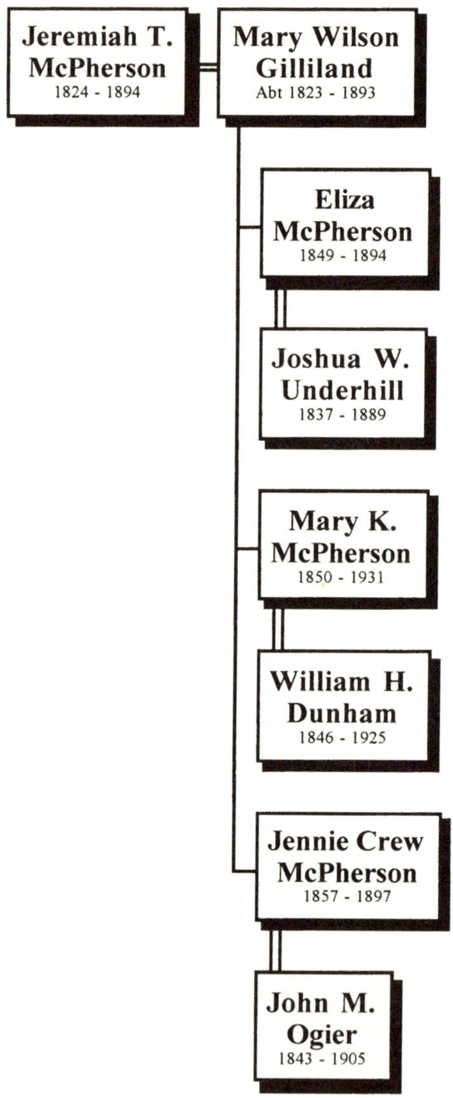

his medical training by spending the 1860-61 year at the Cincinnati College of Medicine and Surgery. Founded in 1851, it was one of the first medical schools to accept females. It continued independently until 1901, when it became part of what is now the College of Medicine at the University of Cincinnati. Rather curiously, according to university records, Underhill only received his degree in 1865, although he must have completed his course work in 1861, since he went in July 1861 to practice in Burnettsville, White County, a settlement of about four hundred in northern Indiana. On the faculty at the medical school had been a father and son, Dr. Robert and Dr. William Spencer, who lived in Monticello, Indiana, only a few miles west of Burnettsville, and they must have encouraged him to settle in the area.

However, the summer of 1861 was not an auspicious time for an unmarried and able-bodied young man to settle down. Hostilities between the North and the South were well underway, and on October 13, 1861, Dr. William Spencer, his medical school teacher and friend, by then Captain William Spencer, enlisted Underhill in Company E of the Indiana 46th Volunteer Infantry Regiment. Two days later, Underhill departed to join his regiment at Logansport, Indiana, relinquishing permanently his practice in Burnettsville.

The Conflict & Early War Years

The tensions in the country that eventually led to the Civil War had existed for some years before Underhill's birth, although during the 1850s, when Underhill was a teenager in Ohio and then trying to get established in his career, they escalated sharply. Since national events directly influenced his life until 1865, a short review may be useful.

The North and the South had developed into quite different cultures. The North had become industrialized, and increasing educational opportunities were producing technical and business people trained to run an industrial economy. The South, however, had remained agrarian, and by comparison to the North, the rate of illiteracy was high. But the South brought in more foreign exchange than the North. The South produced the bulk of the world's cotton supply and over half of the country's exports. Most of the cotton, tobacco, sugar, and rice were obtained through slave labor. While Northerners tended to invest in industry, Southerners tended to invest in land and slaves, a major means of production, and the threat posed by abolition was a loss not only of a way of life but of what Southerners viewed as their private property and their right to do with it as they wished. When the question of slavery came up at a dinner party in Louisiana early in 1860, then Colonel William Tecumseh Sherman observed that "... at the time all men in Louisiana were dreadfully excited on questions affecting their slaves, who constituted the bulk of their wealth, and without whom they honestly believed that sugar, cotton, and rice could not possibly be cultivated."[8]

Overshadowing the other issues that divided the North and the South was slavery, and stemming from that, the question of which region would control the national government. This was not a new issue and had been argued long before Underhill's birth in 1837.

Fifty years earlier, in 1787, the Continental Congress had passed the Northwest Ordinance, establishing the government in the Northwest Territory, the area later to become the states of Ohio, Illinois, Indiana, Michigan, Wisconsin, and part of Minnesota. Slavery was forbidden there as a provision of that ordinance.

Twenty years later, in 1807, the importation of slaves from Africa was banned. In 1820, slavery arose as an issue when Missouri wanted to join the Union at a time when slave and free states were evenly represented in the Senate, thereby upsetting the balance. Many northerners wanted to limit the admission of additional slave states, and ultimately, Henry Clay fashioned what came to be known as the Missouri Compromise. This provided that Missouri would be admitted as a slave state and Maine as a free state, and slavery would be prohibited in the Louisiana Purchase in any new state north of thirty-six degrees thirty minutes north, the southern boundary of Missouri.

In January 1831, six years before Underhill's birth, William Lloyd Garrison, a staunch abolitionist in Boston, issued the first issue of *The Liberator*, and for decades to come, Garrison would vociferously oppose slavery, even becoming too radical for more moderate abolitionists. Boston became a hotbed for abolition, and its promoters were roundly hated in the South.

The Mexican War, during the presidency of James K. Polk, 1845-1849, once again aroused passions over slavery. Polk was a Democrat joined by fellow Democrats in support of the war. The Whigs opposed it. Northerners viewed the war as a means to obtain new land to the south where slavery could be expanded, thereby reinforcing the South's control of the national government. In August 1846, as an amendment to a war appropriations bill, David Wilmot, a first-term representative from Pennsylvania, proposed that slavery be prohibited in any territory acquired from Mexico. Southerners were irate. The House approved the bill but the Congress adjourned before the Senate could vote. In the next session, when the amendment was introduced once again, it was defeated in the Senate and eventually in the House, but for the first time, voting along sectional lines superseded party loyalty.

Polk did not run for a second term. The election of 1848 was won by Zachary Taylor, a revered Mexican War general and a plantation and slave owner who the South felt would be sympathetic to their cause, since the matter of allowing slavery in newly acquired western territories was of paramount concern. As California sought admittance as a free state, tensions between North and South grew high, especially when Taylor, to the chagrin of the South, took the anti-slavery side. Several other issues were involved, and once more, Henry Clay put forth resolutions which he hoped would give both sides something they could accept. The Compromise of 1850 brought in California as a free state, left the matter of slavery in the territories of New Mexico and Utah open, prohibited slave trade, but not slavery, in the District of Columbia, and put teeth into a federal fugitive slave law. But the debate on these issues was heated and painful, and John C. Calhoun feared that if the balance between North and South were destroyed, the South could not with safety remain in the Union.

For anti-slavery forces, the tightening of the fugitive slave law proved galling. Authorities in free states had often turned their backs on enforcing the law, enraging slave owners who wanted assurances they could recover their private property. In an 1842 decision the Supreme Court had ruled that enforcing the fugitive slave law was a federal, not a state, responsibility. Accordingly, a number of free states passed personal liberty laws forbidding the use of state resources in capturing runaway slaves. In several cases in the Northeast during the 1850s, notably in Boston, federal agents seized fugitives despite local efforts to thwart them, so angering local people that many who had been only moderate or indifferent abolitionists found themselves vehement on the issue.

Sectional differences flared sharply once again in 1853 and 1854 over where to run a transcontinental rail line. A southern rail promoter named James Gadsden had become minister to Mexico in order to buy land from Mexico that would allow a line from New Orleans to the Pacific. After negotiations with Mexico and debate in Congress, a land purchase – the so-called Gadsden Purchase – was made. Northerners feared that as a part of this move, attempts would be made to extend slavery into the territories, and they favored a northerly route which would take the line across Kansas and Nebraska.

In order to win Southern support for the northern route, Democratic Senator Stephen Douglas proposed repealing the Missouri Compromise of 1820 and creating two territories, Kansas and Nebraska, where the settlers themselves would decide the issue of slavery. Passage of the Kansas-Nebraska Act in 1854 brought on a bloody conflict in Kansas, where pro-slavery forces battled free soilers for control of the territory. Senator Charles Sumner from Massachusetts was so appalled and disgusted by what was happening that on May 19-20, 1856, he unleashed a vitriolic and pointed attack, largely blaming a pro-slavery faction in Congress for fostering the violence in Kansas. The speech caused an uproar and was widely criticized. Preston Brooks, a congressman from South Carolina, still enraged two days later, assaulted Sumner with a cane so savagely that his injuries kept him out of the Senate for much of the next four years. What enraged the North was not only the attack itself but the southern response, roundly hailing Brooks' action.

Kansas eventually entered the Union in 1861 as a free state, but the bloodshed leading up to it exacerbated growing sectionalism in the Congress, made the schism between North and South almost complete, and essentially destroyed the Whig party. The Republican party emerged from the ruins and Kansas became Republican in reaction to the Democratic pro-slavery forces.

Adding to North-South tension in the decade before the war was the Dred Scott ruling by the Supreme Court in 1857, when Underhill was at Madison College. Dred Scott was a slave taken by his owners into free states but later returned to Missouri. He brought suit in federal court, contending that because he had been taken to free states, where he had resided for extended periods, he should have his freedom. The Court comprised five southern justices, including Marylander Chief Justice Roger B. Taney, and four northern justices, two Democratic and two not. Democratic President Buchanan pressured one of the northern Democratic justices to side with the southern ones. In what northerners saw as an extraordinary decision, Taney ruled that as a Negro, Scott was not considered a U.S. citizen under the Constitution, and therefore was not entitled to sue in federal court; that the Missouri Compromise prohibiting slavery above thirty-six degrees thirty-six minutes was unconstitutional; and furthermore, that Scott had returned to Missouri, a slave state. Pro-slavery forces were delighted by the decision; they felt that Black Republicanism had been knocked on the head. Anti-slavery forces were deeply disturbed, for those same Republicans feared that declaring the Missouri Compromise unconstitutional could open the way for slavery in the northern states.

By the election of 1860, when Underhill was in medical school, the North and South were essentially irreconcilable. The Democrats split hopelessly, unable to agree between North and South upon one candidate. The southern Democrats nominated John Breckinridge, and the northern Democrats nominated Stephen Douglas. Although the Republicans had several possible candidates at their convention in Chicago, Abraham Lincoln presented the fewest drawbacks. The split among the Democrats threw the election to Lincoln, even though he did not run in the South, where he would have stood no chance. In the 1860 election, the control of the country passed to the North, and many in the South felt that their way of life was now directly threatened.

The South had threatened to secede in 1856, but with the tensions that had increased throughout the decade, capped by Lincoln's election, they acted. South Carolina seceded first, on December 20, 1860, followed by Mississippi on January 9, Florida on January 10, Alabama on January 11, Georgia on January 19, Louisiana on January 26, and Texas on February 1. Virginia, Arkansas, North Carolina, and Tennessee adopted a wait-and-see attitude, seceding only late in April and in May after the attack on Fort Sumter. Four border slave states, Missouri, Kentucky, Maryland, and Delaware, did not secede, despite strong secessionist sentiment.

The Confederacy moved quickly to establish its own government. Delegates from the seven seceding states met on February 4, 1861 in Montgomery, Alabama, establishing a government resembling the federal one but with a constitution permitting slavery. Jefferson Davis became President of the Confederate States of America, albeit reluctantly, and Alexander Stephens Vice President. Montgomery remained the Confederate capital only until late May, when it was moved to Richmond, Virginia.

Ironically, many advocating secession did not anticipate war and felt secession would be altogether peaceful. At the time, Colonel W. T. Sherman was serving as the first Superintendent at the newly-formed Louisiana Seminary of Learning and Military Academy, which had opened in January, 1860. After South Carolina seceded, he wrote, "Emissaries came to Louisiana to influence the Governor, Legislature, and people, and it was the common assertion that, if all the Cotton States would follow the lead of South Carolina, it would diminish the chances of civil war, because a bold and determined front would deter the General Government from any measures of coercion."[9]

The Constitution made no provision for secession and was thus no guide under the circumstances. Lincoln had been elected in November, but Buchanan would be a lame duck until March 4. Although elected by strong southern support, Buchanan opposed secession but felt he could in no way coerce a state to remain in the Union. Lincoln was powerless during the lame duck period but made clear his intention to enforce laws. He conceded a right of revolution for justifiable cause but could not accept as a valid justification the lawful election of a president whom one side opposed.

Throughout the early months of 1861, no one knew quite what to do. Some favored action to coerce the return of the secessionists, while others advocated letting them go if they wished. In the end, a take-no-action policy emerged. While Lincoln opposed slavery, he had contended all along that he intended to take no measures to halt it where it existed, since any unionism in the Upper South states was extremely fragile and he wanted if at all possible to keep those states in the Union.

Once secession took place, Confederate officials began negotiating with Union officials for the transfer of federal facilities. In South Carolina, local officials had assured President Buchanan that during negotiations, no hostilities would take place. Fort Sumter, in Charleston harbor, was just being finished as negotiations were in progress, and U.S. troops under their commander, Major Robert Anderson, USA, were stationed at nearby Fort Moultrie. On December 26, 1860 Anderson quietly moved his troops to Fort Sumter. Southerners accused Buchanan of breaking a pledge not to change the military status while negotiations were proceeding, but northerners would not let him crumble under southern pressure and order the troops back to Fort Moultrie. Buchanan tried to get supplies and reinforcements to Anderson, but on January 9, South Carolina fired upon a supply ship, sending it back to sea. Worrying that a war might start imminently, secessionists outside South Carolina urged local officials to step back and allow the Confederacy time to get established.

On March 5, 1861, the day after his inauguration, Lincoln learned that Fort Sumter was running out of provisions. After much deliberation about what action to take so that the North would not appear to provoke a conflict, Lincoln informed South Carolina Governor Francis Pickens that provisions would be sent in, but no reinforcements, as long as the South did not interfere. Rabid secessionists urged Jefferson Davis to take action, asserting that having a Union fort commanding the entrance to Charleston harbor was intolerable and that decisive action would very likely bring Virginia into the Confederacy.

On April 9, the cabinet approved Davis' order. Pierre G. T. Beauregard was to capture the fort before supply ships could get in. A pro forma offer was made to Major Anderson, who refused to surrender, and at 4:30 AM on April 12, firing began on Fort Sumter, the first shots of the Civil War. After a thirty-three hour bombardment, Anderson surrendered.

Lincoln was determined to hold federal facilities and to "enforce laws." On April 15 he issued a proclamation ordering out 75,000 militia for ninety days' service to suppress "combinations too powerful to be suppressed by ordinary causes of judicial proceedings." Each state except for the seceding seven and far western ones was given a quota of regiments to raise, each regiment to "consist on an aggregate of 780 men." Among the several states, Tennessee was asked for 2 regiments; Virginia for 3; North Carolina for 2; Arkansas for 1; Kentucky for 4; Missouri for 4; Delaware for 1; Maryland for 4; Ohio for 13; Illinois for 6; and Indiana for 6. The governors of Tennessee, Virginia, North Carolina, Arkansas, Kentucky, and Missouri flatly refused to comply, in several instances quite sharply, while Ohio and Indiana, as well as other northern states, responded with tumultuous enthusiasm. In Indiana, where Lincoln had requested six regiments, Governor Oliver Perry Morton informed the President that he had raised twelve.

In that spring of 1861, when Underhill was finishing up at medical school in Cincinnati, Washington was in turmoil. The war had broken out just as the new administration was coming in, and throughout the spring, the Washington bureaucracy was upset as both civilian workers and military personnel defected to the Confederacy.

The military on neither side was prepared when the war began. The Confederate military started with a well-trained cadre of officers who had defected and with whatever federal facilities and materiel they could seize but otherwise had to build their forces from scratch. The Union Army comprised 16,000 men spread out over a vast territory, but its officer and enlisted corps shrank as defections occurred. On April 18, General Winfield Scott offered Robert E. Lee command of the Union forces. Lee did not want secession but could not bear to side against his home, and with deep sadness, he resigned from the U.S. Army and returned to Virginia.

In Underhill's home state of Maryland, a slave state, many officials and prominent citizens espoused secession. The Eastern Shore counties were predominantly secessionist, and on March 23, 1863, Underhill noted having heard that his childhood friend Elijah Ward was "going Secesh." Ward had already done so considerably earlier but had joined a unit raised directly by the Confederate States of America, since no Confederate unit could be raised in Maryland. Given its proximity to Washington, Lincoln eventually had to take stiff measures to squelch secessionists there, including suspending habeas corpus, to ensure that Maryland stayed in the Union.

After finishing medical school in the spring, Underhill returned to Fairview, Ohio for a visit. But on July 13, 1861, he left home to begin practicing medicine in Burnettsville, White County, Indiana, a small village even in the modern day, which lies on U.S. 24 about eight miles east of Monticello, the seat of White County, about ten miles west of Logansport, the seat of Cass County, and roughly seventy-five miles north northwest of Indianapolis. As in the rest of Indiana, excitement in White County had run high after Lincoln's April 15th call for troops, and many young men had hastened to enlist.

The first complete organization to enter the service from White County was the Monticello Rifles. They had formed sometime in April, several months before Underhill arrived, and were considerably disappointed early in May when Governor Morton informed them that their services would not be needed, conceivably because Indiana had raised double the number of regiments called for. However, they decided to keep their organization together, and some days later, when the decision was reversed, they were ordered to report to Camp Tippecanoe, in Lafayette, on July 5. The Monticello Rifles became Company K of the Twentieth Regiment, which was organized on July 22 in Indianapolis.[10] Since the ninety-day enlistments from the April call-up expired in July, it was evident that forces would have to be raised to serve for a far longer period. In May Lincoln had authorized recruiting troops for three years, and thus Company K was one of the units called up.

Underhill's unit, Company E of the 46th Indiana, was the next complete outfit from White County to enter the service. On September 30, 1861, Governor Morton authorized Graham N. Fitch and three others to raise a regiment and on that date commissioned the field officers: Graham N. Fitch, Colonel; Newton G. Scott, Lieutenant Colonel; and Thomas H. Bringhurst, Major. On October 7 commissions were granted to Horace Coleman, Surgeon, and to William S. Haymond, Assistant Surgeon, and on December 11 to Robert Irwin, Chaplain, who was later relieved by Hamilton Robb.

Colonel Fitch was a remarkably able man. He was a native of New York but had moved to Logansport in 1843. He was trained as a doctor and for several years was a professor at the Rush Medical College in Chicago. He served in the Indiana legislature and for four years in the U.S. House of Representatives. In 1857 he was elected to the U.S. Senate. He proved a superb commanding officer but had to step down in August 1862 because of an incapacitating injury, at which time Thomas H. Bringhurst relieved him.

Also very able was Assistant Surgeon William S. Haymond, a Renaissance man who was a superb role model for Underhill. Fourteen years older, Haymond had studied medicine and then moved from his native Virginia to Monticello in 1852. He later obtained his degree from the Bellevue Hospital Medical College and became a contributor to medical journals. In addition to being a talented mathematician, he also studied Latin, Greek, French, German, Spanish, and Italian. Although ill health prompted his resignation from the Indiana 46th in December 1862, in 1872 he became president of the Indianapolis, Delphi and Chicago Railroad Company for two years, until he was elected to the U.S. House, where he served on the Committee on Banking and Currency, earning a reputation as its best informed member.

Organization of the 46th Indiana began October 4, and on October 7, barracks at Logansport, paid for by public subscription, were ready. The departure of Underhill's company from Monticello on October 15 seems to have been restrained.

U | 46 | Ind.

Joshua W. Underhill

Pvt, Capt. Spencer's Co., 46 Reg't Ind. Inf.†

Age 23 years.

Appears on

Company Muster-in Roll

of the organization named above. Roll dated

Logansport Ind Nov 5, 1861.

Muster-in to date Nov 5, 1861.

Joined for duty and enrolled:

When Oct 13, 1861.*

Where Burnettsville *

Period .... years.* during War

Bounty paid $ 100 ; due $ 100

Remarks:

† This organization subsequently became Co. E, 46 Reg't Ind. Inf.

* Muster-in roll shows enrollment of all men of this company as of same date, except those enrolled subsequent to date of muster-in of company. See enrollment on subsequent card or cards.

Book mark: 8719. D. 1887

Cameron

(356b) Copyist.

U | 46 | Ind.

Joshua W. Underhill

, Co. E, 46 Reg't Indiana Infantry.

Appears on

Company Descriptive Book

of the organization named above.

DESCRIPTION.

Age 24 years; height 5 feet 11 inches.

Complexion light.

Eyes hazel ; hair dark.

Where born Somerset Co Md.

Occupation Physician

ENLISTMENT.

When Oct 13, 1861.

Where Burnettsville Ind.

By whom Capt Spencer ; term War y'rs.

Remarks: Detached as Hosp Steward Nov 5. 1861.

W. Har. Scott

(888g) Copyist.

Indiana records show that Dr. Joshua W. Underhill was living in Burnettsville, Indiana, when he enlisted into the army on 13 October 1861. He was mustered-in as a Hospital Steward on 5 November 1861.

U | 46 | Ind

J. W. Underhill
Surg. 46 Regt. Ind

Return

of the Post of Lexington, Ky.,
for the month of March, 1865,
dated not dated, 186 ,
shows the following with regard to the person named above:

Post or station
Remarks:

Book mark:

(600) J. F. Maguire Copyist.

U | 46 | Ind

Joshua W Underhill
Surg. 46 Regt. Ind.

Return

of the Post of Lexington, Ky.,
for the month of April, 1865,
dated not dated, 186 ,
shows the following with regard to the person named above:

Post or station
Remarks: Detch'd, Post Surg. Charge of Prisons, Nos. 3 & 4. Lex. Ky.

Book mark:

(600) J. F. Maguire Copyist.

Underhill remained with the 46th Regiment of Indiana Volunteers throughout the war, and in early 1865 he was promoted from Assistant Surgeon to Surgeon. Indiana documents show that he was then stationed with the company at Lexington, Kentucky. By April, the same month that General Lee surrendered at Appomattox and President Lincoln was assassinated, Underhill was Post Surgeon in charge of Prisons Nos. 3 and 4.

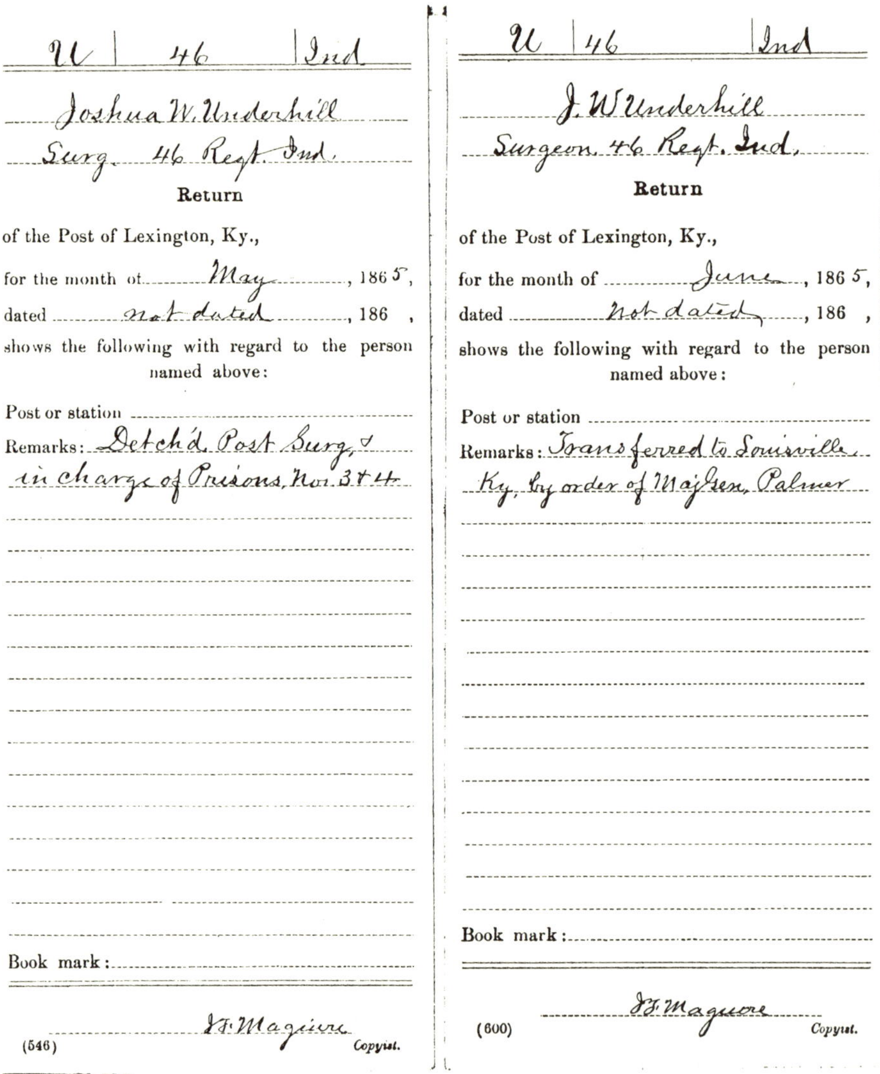

U | 46 | Ind

Joshua W. Underhill

Surg. 46 Regt. Ind.

Return

of the Post of Lexington, Ky.,

for the month of May, 1865,

dated not dated, 186 ,

shows the following with regard to the person named above:

Post or station

Remarks: Detch'd. Post Surg. & in charge of Prisons, Nos. 3 & 4.

Book mark:

J. T. Maguire

(546) Copyist.

U | 46 | Ind

J. W. Underhill

Surgeon. 46 Regt. Ind.

Return

of the Post of Lexington, Ky.,

for the month of June, 1865,

dated Not dated, 186 ,

shows the following with regard to the person named above:

Post or station

Remarks: Transferred to Louisville Ky. by order of Maj Gen. Palmer

Book mark:

(600) J. T. Maguire Copyist.

With the war over, monthly Returns for Underhill show that in June 1865 he was "Transferred to Louisville Ky. By order of Maj Gen. [John M.] Palmer."

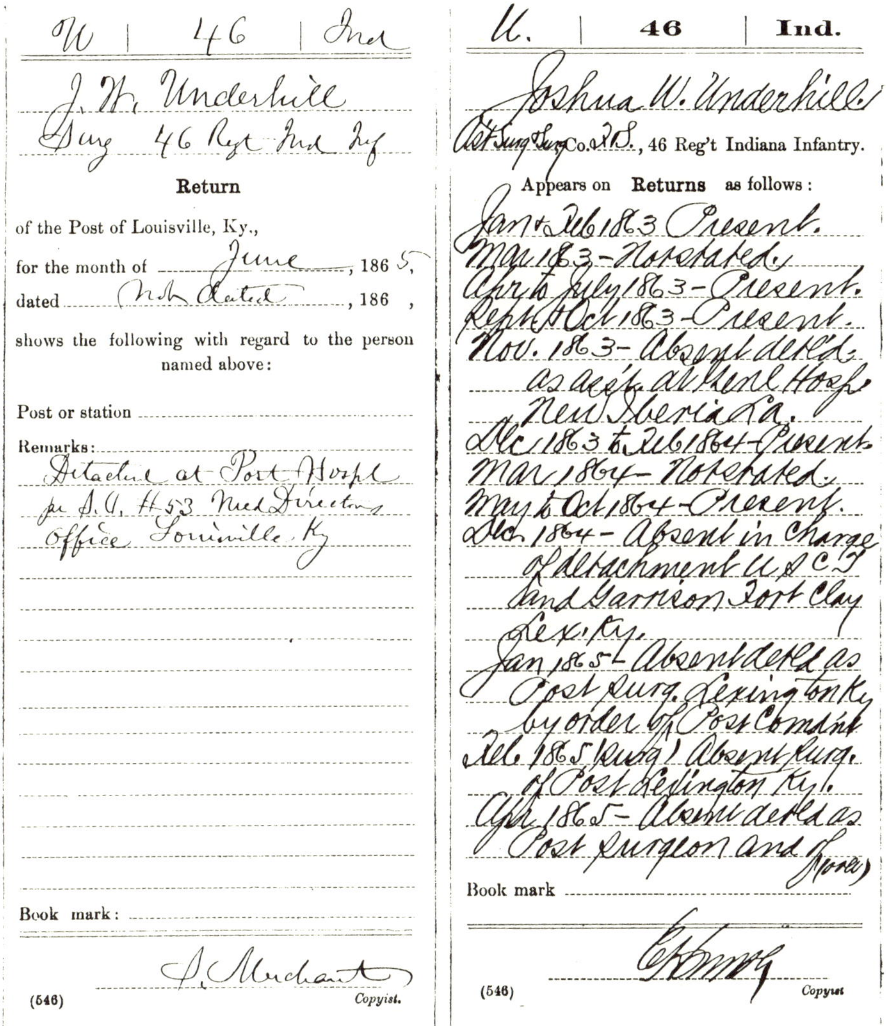

W | 46 | Ind

J. W. Underhill
Surg 46 Regt Ind Inf

Return

of the Post of Louisville, Ky.,
for the month of June, 1865,
dated Not dated, 186 ,
shows the following with regard to the person named above:

Post or station

Remarks: Detached at Post Hospl per S.O. #53 Med Directors Office Louisville Ky

Book mark:

J. Merchant
(546) *Copyist.*

U. | 46 | **Ind.**

Joshua W. Underhill
Ast Surg & Surg, Co. F&S, 46 Reg't Indiana Infantry.

Appears on **Returns** as follows:

Jan & Feb 1863 Present.
Mar 1863 - Not stated.
Apr to July 1863 - Present.
Sept & Oct 1863 - Present.
Nov. 1863 - Absent det'd as ass't at Genl Hosp New Iberia La.
Dec 1863 to Feb 1864 - Present.
Mar 1864 - Not stated.
May to Oct 1864 - Present.
Dec. 1864 - Absent in charge of detachment U.S.C.T. and Garrison Fort Clay Lex. Ky.
Jan 1865 - Absent det'd as Post Surg. Lexington Ky by order of Post Comd't
Feb 1865 (Surg.) Absent, Surg. of Post Lexington Ky.
Apr 1865 - Absent det'd as Post Surgeon and (over)

Book mark

[illegible]
(546) *Copyist*

A Return reviewing Underhill's service since 1863 included entries for his service as an Assistant Surgeon at New Iberia, Louisiana, in November 1863; a December 1864 entry at Fort Clay, Lexington, Kentucky; and the June 1865 Return where he is at the Post Hospital at Louisville, Kentucky.

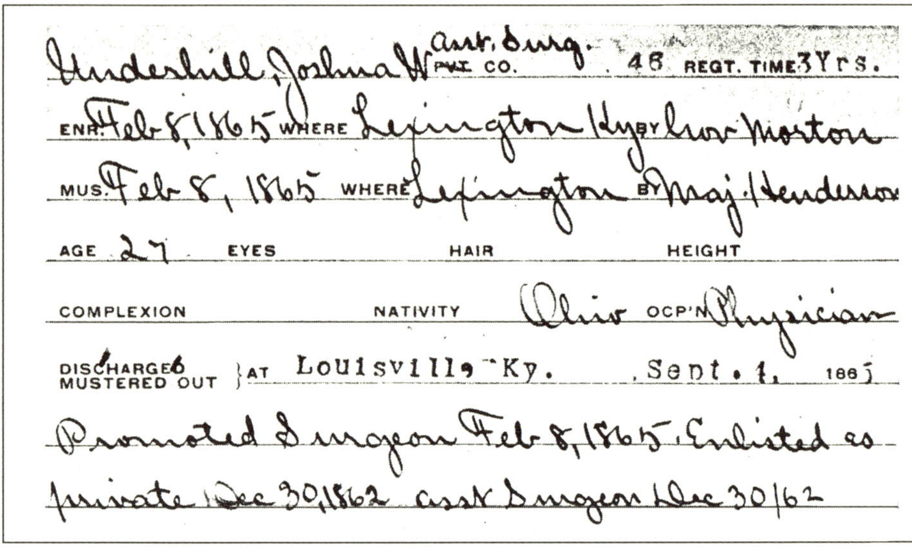
Underhill Joshua W Ass't. Surg. PVT. CO. . 46 REGT. TIME 3 Yrs.
ENR. Feb 8, 1865 WHERE Lexington Ky BY Gov Morton
MUS. Feb 8, 1865 WHERE Lexington BY Maj. Henderson
AGE 27 EYES HAIR HEIGHT
COMPLEXION NATIVITY Ohio OCP'N Physician
DISCHARGED / MUSTERED OUT AT Louisville Ky. Sept. 4, 1865
Promoted Surgeon Feb 8, 1865. Enlisted as private Dec 30, 1862 Asst Surgeon Dec 30/62

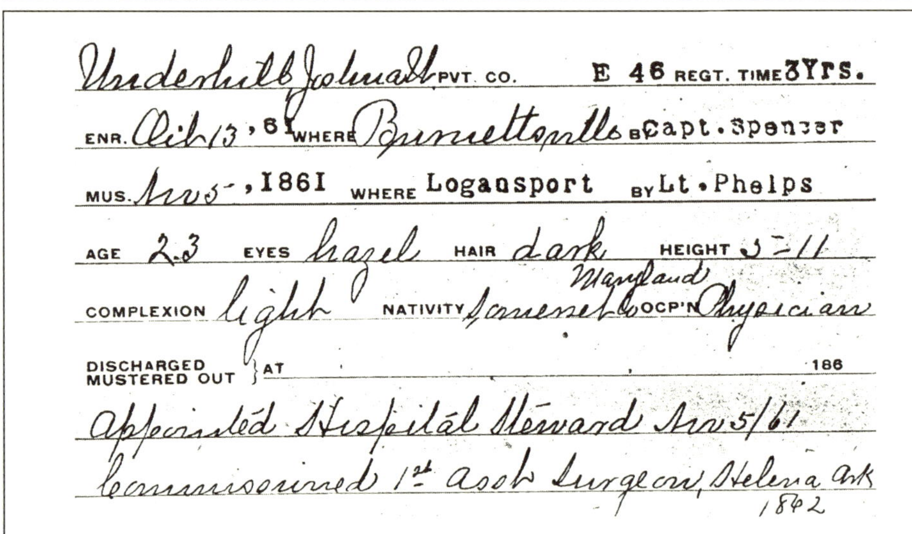
Underhill Joshua W PVT. CO. E 46 REGT. TIME 3 Yrs.
ENR. Oct 13, 61 WHERE Burnettsville BY Capt. Spencer
MUS. Nov 5, 1861 WHERE Logansport BY Lt. Phelps
AGE 23 EYES hazel HAIR dark HEIGHT 5-11
COMPLEXION light NATIVITY Somerset Co Maryland OCP'N Physician
DISCHARGED / MUSTERED OUT AT 186
Appointed Hospital Steward Nov 5/61
Commissioned 1st Asst Surgeon, Helena Ark 1862

Discharge papers for Joshua W. Underhill show his promotion from a Hospital Steward and Private to Assistant Surgeon during his initial three-year enrollment. After his first three-year term, Underhill reenlisted for three more years. He was a Surgeon when he and the rest of his regiment were mustered out of the service on September 4, 1865. His place of nativity is noted incorrectly. It should be Maryland.

> The second complete organization to enter the service from White County was Company E, Forty-sixth Regiment, with Dr. William Spencer, captain; Eli R. Herman, first lieutenant; and Henry Snyder, second lieutenant. These men had pushed the enlistment during the latter part of September and the earlier portion of October, and on the 15th of the latter month the company departed for Logansport to be organized and incorporated into the Forty-sixth Regiment under Graham N. Fitch. Before starting the boys listened to a farewell address from the courthouse steps delivered by T. D. Crow, to which Captain Spencer replied.[11]

On October 15, 1861, at Camp Logan, Logansport, Indiana, Underhill composed a letter to Lazarus Noble, Adjutant General of the Indiana Volunteer Militia:

> Dear Sir:
> At a meeting of our company to day in this camp George W. Spencer was called to the chair & J. W. Underhill appointed secretary, and the following persons declared elected as officers of White Co. "Invincibles."

Captain	–	Will Spencer (M.D.)
1st Lieut.	–	Eli R. Herman
2d "	–	Henry Snyder

> [*A muster roll of the company follows, Underhill including his own name and double underlining M.D. after it.*]

> It is respectfully requested that the commissions may be sent at your earliest convenience.
> Very respt &c.
> George W. Spencer — J. W. Underhill,
> Prest. — sec. of the meeting
> for electing officers.

The Company Muster Roll shows Joshua W. Underhill as having been enrolled by Captain William Spencer as a Private in Company E, 46th Regiment of the Indiana Infantry on October 13, 1861 at Burnettsville, the period of enlistment shown as "during war." He is described in the Company Descriptive Book as age twenty-four, five feet eleven inches tall, with a light complexion, hazel eyes, and dark hair. Remarks note that he detached as Hospital Steward on November 5, 1861, a rank he held until being promoted to Assistant Surgeon on December 30, 1862, upon the resignation of his colleague Dr. Haymond. He was promoted to Surgeon on February 8, 1865, when another colleague, Dr. Israel Washburn, was mustered out. His final rank was noted both as Surgeon and Major.

While Underhill refers often in his diary to Drs. Spencer, Haymond and Washburn, Henry Snyder receives mention only at the back of the diary, where Underhill lists his name with "Expenses of Mess with Capt. Snyder and Lieuts. Spencer and Fisher," but after Underhill's death, Snyder, apparently at the request of Mrs. Underhill, who was applying for a pension, sent an affidavit corroborating her claim that Underhill had been very ill during the war.

Company G formed after Company E and comprising only White County men, also became part of the Indiana 46th. Joseph Cowdin from that company and a county auditor is mentioned in the diary. Company G seems to have received a rather more elaborate send off for Logansport than Company E:

> Company G finally departed from Monticello on the 21st of November, the event being celebrated by a dinner given by the ladies of the town at the house of J. C. Reynolds and ceremonies at the courthouse, which included speeches by Colonel Fitch of the Forty-sixth, Judge Turpie and others, a sword presentation to Captain Sill and a flag presentation to the company.[12]

Both Colonel Fitch and Judge Turpie appear in the diary.

By the time that Underhill's regiment was assembling at Logansport late in 1861, two distinct theaters in the war had developed: the war east of the Appalachians, and the war to the west, where the Indiana 46th would serve. The western theater comprised two parts: the first between the Appalachians and the Mississippi River, the second beyond the Mississippi.

Missouri had refused to send troops for Lincoln's call up in April, but it remained in the Union, despite a large number of secessionists, especially in the southern parts of the state. Throughout middle and late 1861, Confederate and Union forces fought in Missouri but after a series of encounters throughout the state, Union forces managed by January 1862 to force General Price to retreat south to Arkansas.

Kentucky also remained in the Union. Although southern Kentucky was largely secessionist, most of the older population and the legislature were loyal, and Confederates were furious when, in August, Kentuckians elected unionists to the legislature and to Congress. Governor Beriah Magoffin had secessionist sympathies and proclaimed that he wanted to keep the state neutral. Throughout the spring and summer, Lincoln, wanting desperately to keep it in the Union because of its long northern border along the Ohio River, had been scrupulous about their desire for neutrality, although he knew that as a result of his hands-off policy, much materiel reached the Confederacy through Kentucky.

In early September of 1861, however, Kentucky ceased to be neutral. To prevent an anticipated occupation by Federal forces, Confederates under General Leonidas Polk, formerly an Episcopal bishop, occupied Columbus, a town in western Kentucky on the Mississippi River about fifteen miles downstream from Cairo, Illinois. Columbus sits on high bluffs, and to halt river traffic, the Confederates pulled across the river a mile-long chain with links five inches wide, attaching it to two large sycamore trees on the Missouri side and to a six-ton anchor on the other.

Two days after Columbus was seized, General Grant, anticipating a move by General Polk, seized Paducah, on the Ohio River at the mouth of the Tennessee River and ten miles below the mouth of the Cumberland. As well, Kentucky was threatened by two other Confederate forces, one coming from Nashville, under Generals Buckner and Albert Sidney Johnston, and another coming from the Cumberland Gap, under Generals Crittenden and Zollicoffer.

W. T. Sherman, by then a Union brigadier general, had been ordered to Kentucky in late August to serve under now Brigadier General Robert Anderson, the former commanding officer at Fort Sumter. They were to set up their command for the Department of the Cumberland at Louisville. Anderson did not have enough forces to deal with these threats and sent Sherman to the governors of Ohio and Indiana and to General Fremont in St. Louis for more troops. Sherman was unsuccessful.

Brigadier General Anderson had served in the Army for thirty-five years. With the stress of Fort Sumter as well as the fear that his command in Kentucky did not have enough troops to counter the Confederate threat, he soon found the pressure of his job more than he could tolerate, and Sherman was moved up to relieve him. Throughout the fall, Sherman called for more troops, feeling that the critical position of Kentucky was being largely overlooked in Washington. Roughly a month after Sherman's trip to request troops, the 46th Indiana was organized at Logansport.

Underhill's company remained in camp there almost two months, until the regiment was mustered into service. At eight AM on the 12th of December 1861, the men formed up and took the regulation oath, administered by Lieutenant Edgar E. Phelps, USA. Then, accompanied by a band, the regiment marched to the Wabash Railroad depot and boarded a train for Lafayette, Indiana. The *Logansport Journal* of December 14, 1861 describes the scene in heroic language:

> The spectacle was such as has never before been witnessed in this place. The streets through which the regiment marched were crowded with people, and it was

> scarcely possible to make a passage through the mass. The gleam of the bright Enfields, the measured tread of the thousand men, the music, the gallant bearing of the soldiers, and more than all, the thought that all this preparation – this bustle – was, most likely, the opening scene to a bloody tragedy, gave an interest to the occasion that could be experienced at no other time.
>
> * * * * * * * * * * * *
>
> At the depot the scene was still more exciting. No less than four thousand persons had gathered there to take a last look at the boys and bid them good-bye. Mothers who had given up their only son, to subject him to certain hardship, danger, and probably death to vindicate the honor of the Government; fathers bravely struggling against fraternal emotion and exhorting their boys to noble deeds in the defense of the bright; brothers, sisters, husbands, wives, all shaken by a natural grief at the sad parting, yet, with all, not a word of repining, not a wish that the loved ones should remain at home in the hour of their country's peril.[13]

After leaving Lafayette, the regiment went on to Indianapolis, where it remained one night, long enough to receive orders to move on December 14th to Louisville, Kentucky. They took a train from Indianapolis and arrived at Madison, Indiana, on the Ohio River, before dawn the next morning, there embarking on two steamers for Louisville, where they arrived late on the 15th, camping at the Oakland Race Course until the 18th. Then, after several days' marching, the regiment on December 21 reached Bardstown, about sixty miles southwest of Lexington, in the modern day along the Blue Grass Parkway. On Christmas night, 1862, Underhill recorded in his diary, "One year ago to-day was encamped on

Beech Fork of Salt River, near Bardstown, Ky." The weather became bitterly cold, and the men suffered.

After leaving Bardstown on January 6, 1862, the 46th had a cold and muddy twenty-three mile march, arriving in fifteen degree weather at midday on January 7 at Camp Wickliffe, situated in LaRue County, Kentucky, not far from Lincoln's birthplace and named after a former Kentucky governor, Charles Wickliffe. Located on both sides of the road by McDougall's Creek and about five miles east of Hodgenville, in the present day along Highway 270 a little north of Buffalo, Camp Wickliffe was was only in existence from mid-December 1861 to mid-February 1862 and served as an assembly camp for Union regiments. Where the camp was located is now private property with nothing to indicate it was ever there. That winter at Camp Wickliffe was miserable. The weather was wet and cold, the troops drilled three hours every afternoon, and discipline was harsh.

But February 1862 brought significant Union gains in Kentucky and Tennessee. In January, Confederate forces suffered defeats in Kentucky. In early February, Brigadier General Ulysses S. Grant and Naval Commodore Andrew H. Foote took Fort Henry, on the Tennessee River in Tennessee, just south of the Kentucky border, with combined land and naval forces. After a much more difficult battle on February 16, 1862, again using land and naval forces, Grant captured Fort Donelson, on the Cumberland River in Tennessee, ten miles east of Fort Henry. The victories at Forts Henry and Donelson owed much to the naval forces involved, and Underhill mentions many of the vessels.

At the outbreak of war in April 1861, the U.S. Navy was a sea-going force only, with no capacity or authority for river warfare. General Fremont in St. Louis had initiated construction of a naval fleet on the Mississippi. James Eads (1820-1887), a boat builder at St. Louis, oversaw a crash building program of seven ironclad gunboats—designated city-class because they were named after river ports—which were commissioned in January 1862. Designed by Samuel Pook, they were

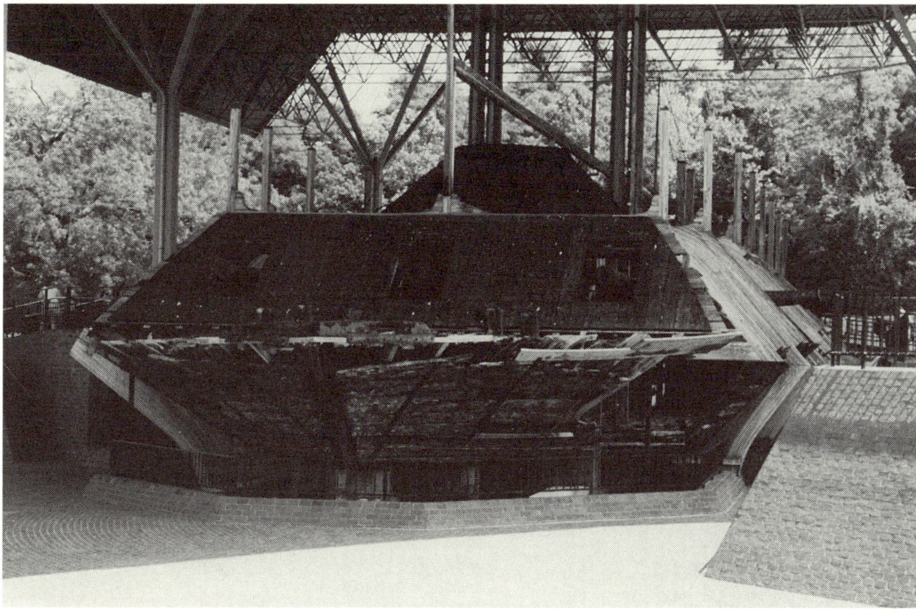

The U.S.S. *Cairo* was one of seven ironclad "city class" gunboats (each named after river port-cities such as Cairo, Illinois, and Mound City, Illinois) that were commissioned in January 1862. Sunk in the Yazoo River 12 December 1862, the *Cairo* was raised in the 1960's and is now displayed at the Vicksburg Military Park.

dubbed "Pook's Turtles" because of their unusual design. Flat bottomed and low in the water, they were 175 feet long with a 51 foot beam, carried thirteen guns and were designed to fight bow on. Heavy iron plating over thick laminated wood protected the machinery and the crew's quarters. They were: the *Louisville;* the *Cincinnati;* the *St. Louis,* on October 12, 1861 the first to be launched and later renamed the *Baron De Kalb;* the *Pittsburg;* the *Carondelet,* after Carondelet, Missouri, then a small town on the Mississippi about ten miles south of St. Louis with a marine railway but after 1870 a neighborhood of St. Louis; the *Cairo,* named after Cairo, Illinois, the town at the junction of the Ohio and Mississippi Rivers, watched for in the night by Mark Twain's Huck and

Jim, so they could take a steamboat into free territory; and the *Mound City,* after Mound City, Illinois, a town about seven miles upstream on the Ohio River from Cairo. Four were built at Carondelet: the *Carondelet,* which was constructed in forty-five days; the *Louisville,* the *St. Louis,* and the *Pittsburg.* The *Mound City,* the *Cincinnati,* and the *Cairo* were built at Mound City, where remnants of the marine railway can still be seen.

Although stout, "Pook's Turtles" were not invulnerable. On many occasions they were hit and put out of action, even sunk, temporarily, but given the technology of the day, they seem to have been relatively easy to repair. Underhill mentions all but the *Cairo,* but this is not surprising, since by the time he makes his first reference to a city-class gunboat, the *Cairo* had been on the bottom of the Yazoo River for just over a month. During the war, it was the only one to sink and not be recovered. On December 12, 1862, the *Cairo* and two other boats were twelve miles up the Yazoo River reconnoitering for places to land troops for an assault on Vicksburg when she hit an undetected Confederate torpedo, or mine, and went down in twelve minutes. Her smokestacks remained sticking up above the water, and the next day, Admiral David D. Porter, Commander of the Mississippi Squadron, fearing she might be raised, destroyed this evidence. Because of this, not until 1964 was she found and raised off the bottom. Her remains can be seen today in the Vicksburg Military Park. Ironically, she is the only surviving example, since soon after the war, several were scrapped and at least two sank.

Twice as large as the seven city-class ironclads was the *Benton,* a gunboat with sixteen guns, used by Commodore Foote as his flagship. She had originally been a snag boat (a steamboat with apparatus designed to catch debris in the water) but was converted to an iron-clad. The *Essex, Tyler, Conestoga,* and *Lexington* were partially clad, the *Essex* having been a ferry that was remodeled and fitted up as a gunboat. As well, thirty-eight mortar boats were constructed at St. Louis and taken down to Cairo for armaments. They had no power and were towed by steamers, but the mortars on board could throw a shell several miles.

At first, river operations came under Army command – the Army had contracted for the city-class gunboats – but the motley crews that manned the vessels were under the command of naval officers. Only in the fall of 1862 did the Navy take over the river squadrons, but fortunately, Grant and Foote worked together extremely well, because the river fleet played a major part in regaining control of the Mississippi River.

The Mississippi and its tributaries drain thirty-one states. Because of acts of God and nature and the U.S. Army Corps of Engineers, many changes have taken place since the Civil War. But at that time, the river system comprised some 17,000 miles of waterways, largely navigable by steamboat, depending on the season of the year. In the spring, water levels tended to rise with the winter melt-off but to drop later in the year, making some waterways unnavigable. In 1811, the first Mississippi steamboat, the *New Orleans,* appeared on the river, and over six thousand would be built by the end of the century. They transformed life and trade along the river, and by the outbreak of the Civil War, passenger and freight service was well established, as were connections to rail. Especially in the days before good road transport and extensive railroad development, the river system served as a critically important transportation artery vital both to northern and southern states in its watershed.

In the lower Mississippi, larger towns along the river became important depots for cotton and sugar. Because of frequent lowland flooding, these towns were often located on bluffs, which provided excellent locations for fortifications and guns, allowing towns to be defended easily from river attack. Control of the Mississippi gave the Confederacy freedom to move men and materiel wherever they wished on the river.

Early in the war, Washington had decided to choke the Confederacy by throwing up a naval blockade so that nothing could move in or out of Southern seaports. Opening up the Mississippi would allow the North to wage war deep into the Confederacy, keep its products from reaching seaports, and cut off its western states. Regaining contol of

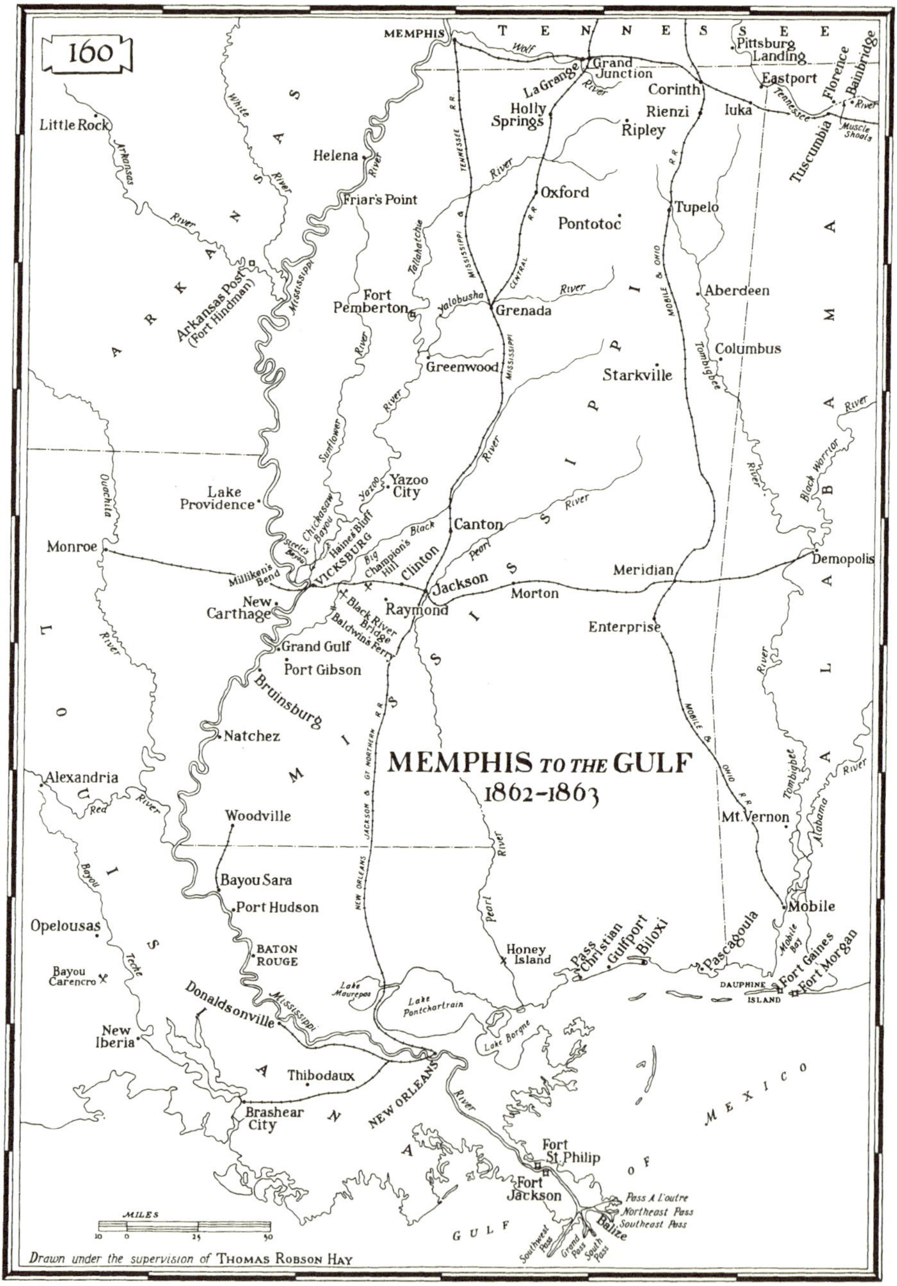
160
MEMPHIS TO THE GULF
1862-1863
MEMPHIS
TENNESSEE
ARKANSAS
MISSISSIPPI
ALABAMA
LOUISIANA
GULF OF MEXICO
Little Rock
Helena
Friar's Point
Arkansas Post (Fort Hindman)
Fort Pemberton
Greenwood
Grenada
Holly Springs
La Grange
Grand Junction
Corinth
Rienzi
Ripley
Iuka
Pittsburg Landing
Eastport
Florence
Bainbridge
Tuscumbia
Muscle Shoals
Oxford
Pontotoc
Tupelo
Aberdeen
Columbus
Starkville
Lake Providence
Yazoo City
Canton
Milliken's Bend
Steele's Bayou
Chickasaw Bayou
Haines Bluff
VICKSBURG
Big Champion's Hill
Clinton
Jackson
Morton
Meridian
Demopolis
Monroe
New Carthage
Raymond
Black River Bridge
Baldwins Ferry
Enterprise
Grand Gulf
Port Gibson
Bruinsburg
Natchez
Alexandria
Woodville
Mt. Vernon
Bayou Sara
Port Hudson
Opelousas
Mobile
BATON ROUGE
Bayou Carencro
Honey Island
Pass Christian
Gulfport
Biloxi
Pascagoula
Fort Gaines
Fort Morgan
DAUPHINE ISLAND
Mobile Bay
Donaldsonville
Lake Maurepas
Lake Pontchartrain
Lake Borgne
New Iberia
Thibodaux
NEW ORLEANS
Brashear City
Fort St. Philip
Fort Jackson
Pass A L'outre
Northeast Pass
Southeast Pass
Balize
Southwest Pass
Grand Pass
South Pass
Mississippi
White River
Arkansas River
Wolf River
Tennessee River
Tallahatchie
Yalobusha
Sunflower
Yazoo
Black
Pearl River
Ouachita
Red River
Bayou Teche
Tombigbee River
Black Warrior River
Alabama River
MISSISSIPPI & TENNESSEE R.R.
MISSISSIPPI CENTRAL R.R.
MOBILE & OHIO R.R.
NEW ORLEANS JACKSON & GT NORTHERN R.R.
MILES
10 0 25 50
Drawn under the supervision of THOMAS ROBSON HAY

the river became a strategic Union objective, therefore, and from late winter 1862 until mid July 1863, the 46th Indiana was involved in that campaign.

On February 14, 1862, the 46th Indiana left Camp Wickliffe, marching in very cold weather over bad roads to the mouth of the Salt River, on the Ohio, very close to West Point, Kentucky, which they reached on the 17th. There Underhill's company embarked on the *Golden State*, Major Bringhurst the field officer aboard. Although the reason is not disclosed in the regimental history, their subsequent move to Paducah may have resulted from Grant's plan of late February to move on Columbus, with Foote's fleet. This, however, proved unnecessary. After the Confederate losses at Forts Henry and Donelson, Beauregard ordered Polk to abandon Columbus, and on March 4, Union forces took permanent possession.

Underhill, however, had not marched with his regiment when it left Camp Wickliffe. He had been on detached duty as surgeon with the 15th Indiana Infantry. In his March 4, 1863 diary entry, he notes almost casually his subsequent odyssey in search of his outfit: "One year ago to-day was in Nashville, Tennessee. Arrived there on 26th of February just two days after its surrender to the Federals. Staid there till about the 8th. Had been left at Cp. Wickliffe, Ky in charge of our sick and started on search of Regt 17th of Feby, found it one month afterwards at New Madrid, Missouri."

Simultaneous with the 46th's departure from Camp Wickliffe, a force of about 25,000 troops to be called the Army of the Mississippi was being assembled above Cairo on the west bank of the Mississippi River under Major General John Pope for the purpose of moving with naval forces against the Confederates who had fallen back to New Madrid and Island No. 10 after abandoning Columbus. After leaving Paducah, the 46th continued by steamers, on February 23 joining General Pope's army at Commerce, Missouri, on the Mississippi River forty miles north of New Madrid. From there it marched south, to the rear of New Madrid, where Underhill eventually rejoined his unit.

After having to abandon Columbus, Kentucky, the Confederates had withdrawn both to Island No. 10 – so designated because of its being the tenth island in the Mississippi south of the confluence with the Ohio River – and to New Madrid, Missouri. Island No. 10 was about fifty river miles downstream from Columbus, New Madrid another ten. New Madrid, sitting at the top of a large horseshoe bend in the river, had been heavily fortified with guns and was occupied by five Confederate regiments and several artillery companies. Six gunboats on the river added to the defenses. General Pope decided to attack New Madrid first, but while he was waiting for large guns to arrive, he established a battery at Point Pleasant, some twelve miles downstream, to cut off the Confederates from supplies coming upriver, thus forcing Brigadier General John P. McCown, the Confederate general commanding at New Madrid, to get reinforcements from Island No. 10 upstream. By March 13, Pope's heavy guns had arrived from Cairo, and he began a bombardment. By that night it was evident to McCown that further resistance was useless, and leaving behind unburied dead and most of their equipment, the Confederates fled upstream to Island No. 10.

While the rest of the Union force pursued them, Underhill's regiment along with three others moved downstream some fifteen miles along the Missouri shore to Riddle's Point to install a battery across from Tiptonville, Tennessee, where the Confederates had forces that could communicate with Island No. 10, five or six miles away.

On March 18-19, the troops worked virtually all night constructing the battery and early the next morning, fired upon two transports headed upstream. With this, four Confederate gunboats crossed from Tiptonville and fired upon the emplacement for an hour and a quarter without managing to inflict heavy casualties or to dislodge the troops.

Meanwhile, the attack now focused on Island No. 10. With Union forces occupying New Madrid, the river south was effectively blockaded, and upstream the Union had control. On March 15, a gunboat fleet from Cairo under Commodore Foote with eight gunboats, ten mortar boats, and two infantry regiments arrived several miles upstream of Island No. 10, and the next day a bombardment began which lasted until April 7. Shortly thereafter, the Confederates withdrew, but not before three generals, over a hundred siege guns, artillery, and other arms were captured, along with 6700 prisoners. This action was simultaneous with the Battle of Shiloh, at Pittsburg Landing, Tennessee which the Union won, albeit with heavy casualties on both sides, and where the Confederates lost General Albert Sidney Johnston. On April 9, after Island No. 10 had fallen, Underhill's regiment left Riddle's Point and crossed the river on the side-wheel packet *Ohio Belle* to Tiptonville.

Leaving Tiptonville on April 13, 1862, the 46th Indiana started south by water with a large force under General Pope for Fort Pillow, which lay on the Tennessee shore of the Mississippi about seventy miles north of Memphis. It was situated on the First Chickasaw Bluff, which rose up to one hundred feet and was the first good position for defense below Island No. 10. Given bends in the river, the fort commanded a view of several miles up and downstream. On the 16th, the twenty-two transports tied up at Osceola, on the Arkansas side just above Fort Pillow. On April 17, however, General Henry W. Halleck, commanding the Department of the Mississippi, suddenly changed his mind, ordering General Pope and most of his forces to Pittsburg Landing. Accordingly, twenty of the transports went back upstream, leaving behind with Commodore Foote only a small force of 1200 men, the 43rd and 46th Indiana regiments, under Colonel Fitch, commander of the 46th, aboard the *Graham* and the *Emma.*

The Union paid a high price for Halleck's decision. Grant felt that taking Vicksburg would have been far easier had the Union made its attempt immediately following the Battle of Shiloh. Underhill makes a similar observation in his April 13, 1863 diary entry, when he comments that "...We are one year too late in our attempts to take Vicksburg."

In part, a cumbersome Union command structure was to blame. Grant observed that Albert Sidney Johnson was effectively in command of all Confederate forces west of the Appalachians, whereas the Union had created four separate commands in that theater without one general in a position to take charge of them all. Only after the Battle of Shiloh did General Halleck come from St. Louis to assume command of the combined armies. He deemed Corinth, Mississippi, a rail junction just south of the Tennessee border, a more important objective for the moment, and as a result, the Union missed a splendid opportunity to seize Vicksburg.

At Forts Henry and Donelson and at New Madrid and Island No. 10, the formula for victory had been a large land force attacking from the rear in addition to bombardment from the gunboats. After Pope's departure, however, Colonel Fitch's force was too small to take Fort Pillow. As well, Foote was faced with nine Confederate gunboats already at the fort, with others reportedly en route, although the nine did not worry him especially since despite their heavy guns, the boats were wooden. What was worrying Foote increasingly was painful swelling resulting from a serious ankle wound sustained from heavy flying splinters while aboard the *St. Louis* when it was hit at Fort Donelson, and early in May, he asked to be relieved, relinquishing command of the Western Gunboat Flotilla to Captain C. H. Davis.

Foote had under his command ten mortar boats and eight gunboats, seven iron-clad. On April 17, the same day Halleck recalled Pope, Foote began bombarding Fort Pillow and the Confederate gunboats, without much effect. By May 10, Davis was in command when a Confederate naval force attacked. Eight Confederate ironclad rams attacked the mortar boats. In the battle, the *Cincinnati* and the *Mound City* were put out of action temporarily. Two Confederate boats were disabled, and the engagement broke off after an hour.

Meanwhile, during the five weeks until Fort Pillow was evacuated on June 4, the men of the Indiana 43rd and 46th simply had to wait. The troops were ashore by day and on the transports by night. Because of high water in the river, the ground at Osceola was wet. The weather was sweltering, and half of the men were sick. On April 23 the list unfit for duty numbered 104. At this time, Underhill became very ill with malaria and chronic diarrhea and later alleged that he had ended up on a hospital boat for four months. His colleague, Dr. Israel Washburn, commented that Underhill also had the worst case of jaundice he had ever seen.

What finally effected the evacuation of Fort Pillow were defeats the Confederates had suffered elsewhere in Tennessee. Their forces at Fort Pillow would have been virtually cut off had they remained. There had been rumors from the end of May that the Confederates were soon to leave, but on the night of June 4, the Confederates set fire to whatever would burn, and very early the next morning, the fort was found to be empty. The Indiana 43rd and 46th regiments raised their flags over the fort, and on that same afternoon, they headed downstream for Memphis.

At Memphis, on June 6, the Western Gunboat Flotilla engaged in a two-hour gunboat fight. Excited crowds lined the bluffs to watch the contest, and the concussion from a Union ram colliding at fifteen knots with a Confederate boat was felt on the shore. Five Union ironclads and two rams successfully demolished seven of eight Confederate boats. The *History of the Forty-Sixth Regiment Indiana Volunteer Infantry* notes rather wryly that while some hundred Confederate sailors were being fished from the water by their opponents, "a band on one of the boats played 'Dixie' for the comfort of the shivering rebels."[14] The mayor of Memphis immediately surrendered, and as Underhill reminisced in a June 6, 1863 entry, "One year ago to-day we took possession of Memphis. The 43rd and 46th Ind- Regiments constituted all the Infantry. City surrendered after a severe gunboat fight in which almost the entire Rebel flotilla was destroyed."

Colonel Fitch of the 46th Indiana took firm control. He sent Major Bringhurst across the river to Hopefield, Arkansas, the eastern terminus of the Memphis & Little Rock Railroad, where several guns, locomotives, and much railroad iron were captured. Fitch also met with Memphis city officials, allowing them to continue in office while the military undertook to enforce federal law. The regiment remained in

Memphis until June 15. It then boarded the side-wheel *New National*, captured in Memphis, to go up the White River in Arkansas to meet the army of General Samuel Curtis coming from Missouri.

While Halleck had been directing operations for the move on Corinth, Mississippi, which had prevented Pope's army from advancing down the river to Vicksburg, Union General Samuel R. Curtis had been fighting in Arkansas, in the trans-Mississippi theater. By the end of 1861, Confederate forces had been forced out of southern Missouri and into Arkansas. Early in 1862, Confederate General Earl Van Dorn took command of the trans-Mississippi Department, and at Pea Ridge, Arkansas, his forces and Curtis' clashed in March 1862. The Confederates were routed. Van Dorn's scattered forces withdrew south and Curtis went north into southern Missouri. In May, Curtis returned to Arkansas by a more easterly route, going to Batesville on the White River, from which he had wanted to move on Little Rock, some eighty miles southwest, whose federal arsenal had been seized by the Confederates in 1861, even before secession. Although the need by both sides for forces in Tennessee prevented either from prosecuting an aggressive campaign in Arkansas, the 46th Indiana went on an expedition up the White River in June 1862, after leaving Memphis, to open communications with Curtis' forces. The White River, navigable for a considerable distance, flows roughly south through Arkansas, emptying into the Mississippi a few miles above Napoleon, a town about fifty miles below Helena at the mouth of the Arkansas River and no longer there. On June 17, at St. Charles, Arkansas, the 46th found itself in a spirited engagement.

Underhill refers twice to the June 17 fight at St. Charles, and at the end of the diary, he introduces a poem about this battle with the following comment:

> The following lines were written for a New York illustrated paper on the fight at St. Charles, White River, Ark's, on June 17th, 1862. The 46th Ind. was only

> Infantry engaged – the gunboats were the "Cincinnati," "Carondelet," "Lexington" and the ill-fated "Mound City." A 64 pound shot, penetrating the Mound City, cut the connecting pipe, whereupon every portion of the boat was filled with hot steam, scalding to death the entire crew of about 175 – except some 25 who were slightly burned.

Men plunged into the river, only to drown or be shot at by Confederates along the shore. There the river is perhaps a tenth of a mile across, and with substantial growth up to the water's edge, lines of sight are limited and hidden batteries would have been hard to detect. A marker at the site today carries these words:

> Here on June 17, 1862 a Federal fleet of eight vessels attempted to force its way upstream past Confederate shore defenses commanded by Captain Joseph Fry. The Confederates disabled the Union gunboat *Mound City* with heavy casualties before their positions were overrun by troops of the Forty-sixth Indiana Volunteers. The cannon shot which put the *Mound City* out of action has been described as the most destructive single shot fired in the Civil War.

After several weeks more along the White River, where they eventually encountered General Curtis' forces, the regiment left St. Charles on July 14 for Helena, Arkansas, where it was assigned to General Hovey's division. The Indiana 46th was based at Helena from mid-July 1862 until its departure for Vicksburg the following April.

Helena

Helena was occupied by the army of Union General Samuel R. Curtis at the end of June 1862, and by the fall, it had become a major Union staging base and supply depot for the Vicksburg campaign. In Phillips County, Arkansas, Helena lies on the west bank of the Mississippi River about sixty river miles south of Memphis and forty-five miles north of the mouth of the White River. In the 1860 census, Phillips County had 8817 slaves, 3558 adult white males and 2465 adult white females. Helena was a substantial town with many lovely houses and many stores, in one of which Underhill bought his diary. It was an important river port where mule trains would bring cotton for shipment to New Orleans.

The Helena riverfront has changed greatly since 1862. In the aftermath of severe flooding in 1927, a big levee was constructed along the river bank, making the river invisible from the town, but at the time of the war, the town for half a mile or so back from the Mississippi was essentially flat and extended inland from the river six blocks and was eight blocks long. Behind the town lie steep ridges, part of what is called Crowley's Ridge. Just behind the town, on a much lower ridge, was Fort Curtis, named for General Samuel R. Curtis, and dedicated October 30, 1862, as Underhill notes in his diary, which he had started only a few days before. In September of 1862, General Curtis was assigned to the command of the Department of the Missouri, General Frederick Steele succeeding him at Helena. General B. M. Prentiss, whom Underhill describes in detail in a March 15, 1863 entry, then relieved Steele and was commander at the time of a Confederate attack in July 1863. No traces of Fort Curtis remain in Helena today except for an historical marker on Perry Street showing where it stood.

The Union had gained increasing control of the river system in 1862. Victories at Forts Henry and Donelson opened the Tennessee and Cumberland rivers. Following the Confederate exodus, Columbus, Kentucky became a major Union supply depot. More victories followed, at New Madrid, Island No. 10, Fort Pillow, and Memphis. Late in April, Admiral David G. Farragut took New Orleans, and during May and June he moved upriver, forcing Baton Rouge and Natchez to surrender. The Union naval pincers were getting closer to each other. But a June 1862 attempt to take Vicksburg failed after Farragut encountered blistering gunfire from the highly fortified "Gibraltar of the West" and after a request to General Halleck for supporting troops was denied. After the CSS *Arkansas* crippled the USS *Carondelet,* Farragut retreated south, the river gunboats went back to Helena, and the Confederacy still retained control over more than two hundred river miles of the Mississippi, from Port Hudson, Louisiana on the south to Vicksburg on the north. Conquering Vicksburg would take another year.

Lincoln wanted Vicksburg. "Let us get Vicksburg and all that country is ours," he urged. " The war can never be brought to a close until that key is in our pocket." Almost all of Underhill's diary deals with the period while that was being achieved.

Vicksburg, Mississippi lies at and below a fishhook curve in the Mississippi, at the time of the Civil War about seven miles downstream from the mouth of the Yazoo River. Across from Vicksburg on the peninsula at DeSoto, Louisiana, was the eastern terminus of the Shreveport railroad. Vicksburg was the western terminus of the railroad from Jackson, the state capital some forty-five miles east.

After the Union missed its chance early in 1862 to seize Vicksburg, the Confederates fully availed themselves of the opportunity to fortify the city of five thousand, placing for several miles along its high bluffs guns that could rake any passing vessel with murderous fire, especially an upstream boat struggling against a four knot current. The steep bluffs made a land assault from the river virtually impossible.

In late June 1862, Brigadier General Thomas Williams embarked on a scheme to get around Vicksburg. He supervised the digging of a canal across the peninsula some distance back from the city with the hope that it would change the channel of the river, allowing vessels to bypass the guns of Vicksburg altogether. But his men were succumbing to heat and to malaria, the level of the river was dropping, and after the canal's completion, the Confederates chortled when the Mississippi refused to go where it was wanted.

By late fall of 1862, any hopes that the war would end shortly had been dashed, and morale in the North had plummeted. General Grant, deeply worried by this, felt it imperative do whatever possible to take Vicksburg. In a day when armies tended to go into camp during winter months, Grant felt idleness would ruin the spirit and conditioning of his troops. Thus, between the time the 46th Indiana arrived at Helena in July 1862 until its departure in April 1863, he made several attempts to take Vicksburg, recognizing that although some had a poor chance of succeeding, they would keep his troops active. Since Helena was an important staging area for Union troops, Underhill was able to observe and report on troop movements along the river, most of them connected with Vicksburg. Although Underhill spent nearly all that period in Helena, the rest of the regiment was involved in some of these operations as well as several others.

One of the first operations that engaged the 46th was a move against Arkansas Post. Settled in 1686, Arkansas Post was one of the earliest European communities in the lower Mississippi Valley. Its population was greatest when it was the capital of Arkansas but declined after the capital was moved to Little Rock in 1821. It lay on the north side of the Arkansas River, which flows roughly southeast through Arkansas draining a few miles beyond into the Mississippi. Grant estimates the distance at fifty miles, Sherman at forty, perhaps because the fleet first went up the White River and then into the

Arkansas through a cutoff. Fort Hindman at Arkansas Post was held by five thousand men under the Confederate General T. J. Churchill. On November 16, 1862, Underhill documents the 46th's departure on an expedition against the Post:

> This (Sunday) morning an expedition started for some point unknown down the Mississippi. Gen Hovey's division about 7,000 troops under command of Gen. Washburn 14 steamers laden with troops, took rations for 10 days and expect to return. No one allowed to pass pickets since order for expedition given. I am left in charge of 35 sick the hospital portion of which will be seen by Dr. Lyons of 24th Iowa...."

On November 20, he writes, "Last night returned the *Gladiator* from the expedition. Came for 10 days more provisions. Reports leaving the fleet at the mouth of the White River."

On November 22, his entry was longer:

> Last night expedition returned. Their destination was Arkansas Post on the Arkansas River about 8 miles from its mouth. The intention was to proceed up White River a short distance perhaps to Prairie Landing and from thence march across to the Post. The White was found too low to allow the passage of the boats. Owing to the swamps with which the country abounds about the mouth of the White it was impossible to make the march from that point or from the mouth of the Arkansas. Therefore after making every reasonable attempt it was found impossible to proceed and the expedition was compelled to return. It has been ascertained that Arkansas Post has been pretty well fortified and is garrisoned by 5,000 Secesh. They therefore have

> command of the Arkansas at that point. Whether another attempt will be made to dislodge them is not yet certain.

In late November, Underhill observed another expedition taking shape that involved the 46th. General Sherman writes that he had been summoned for a conference with General Grant, who wanted to make an advance south in Mississippi and wanted General Curtis

> ...to send an expedition from some point on the Mississippi near Helena, ...toward Grenada, to the rear of Pemberton [Lt. Gen. John C. Pemberton, Confederate general commanding the Army of Mississippi which included the garrison at Vicksburg], it would alarm him for the safety of his communications, and would assist us materially in the proposed attack on his front....I dispatched my aide...to Helena, who returned, bringing me a letter from General Frederick Steele, who had just reached Helena with Osterhaus's division, and who was temporarily in command, General Curtis having gone to St. Louis. This letter contained the assurance that he "would send from Friar's Point a large force under Brigadier-General A. P. Hovey in the direction of Grenada, aiming to reach the Tallahatchie at Charleston, on the next Monday, Tuesday, or Wednesday (December 1st) at furthest." My command was appointed to start on Wednesday, November 24th....[15]

On November 20, Underhill had written, " Rumored that Steele's and Osterhaus' divisions are returning for this point via the Mississippi River." On November 22, he confirmed it: " Gen. Steele and Osterhaus are returning. Their advance came in by the river this afternoon." On November 25, Underhill writes, "Rumors are to day that another expedition leaves down the river with 20 days' rations tomorrow." On November 27th Underhill notes, "The rumored expedition left this afternoon but to what point is not known. They went down the river. The force consisted of perhaps ten thousand infantry, cavalry, and artillery. The last expedition instead of being commanded by Washburn was under Gen. Hovey." The 46th Indiana accompanied the expedition down the Tallahatchie and Coldwater Rivers.

Underhill reports December 5 on the results of the expedition: "Rumors rec'd that some cavalry of the expedition that left on the 27th inst. had a skirmish also that at another time our boys captured a number of cars and cannon and tore up the R. R. from Grenada to Memphis. Rumored, too, that they will return in a few days."

By December 7, they had. On that day he writes:

> Expedition returned to day Sunday. They proceeded across the R. R. from Grenada to Memphis, to the Ohio and Mississippi R. R. both of which roads they destroyed for some distance, burning several important bridges and destroying the tracks for some distance. Thus Price's communication to the rear is cut off. The expedition having accomplished the object for which it was sent out returned to day having lost a few men by bushwhacking. A few prisoners were brought in. Our cavalry were within five miles of Grenada.

The expedition had succeeded in getting Pemberton to give up the Tallahatchie.

After this foray, Grant made an attempt at Vicksburg. He would lead a major movement south through Mississippi and directed Sherman to take a force by steamer and with the cooperation of the naval forces, to go up the Yazoo River and land in the vicinity of Vicksburg and to take the city by whatever means he thought proper. Grant was to hold Pemberton's force away from Vicksburg to the north but was to follow and back up Sherman if Pemberton retreated to Vicksburg. Sherman began this expedition from Memphis, and on December 21, 1862 at Helena, Underhill saw this taking form. The 46th did not go.

> This morning a large number of transports arrived loaded with troops – been coming all day – 72 are said to be here and on the route two divisions of this army, Steele's and Washburn's Cavalry Division it is said will also accompany the expedition. This will swell the number of troops to at least sixty thousand. Vicksburg is thought to be the point of attack. Six Ohio Regts 14th, 16th, 42nd, 54th, 114th, and 120th I have seen to day.... Gen. Sherman commands the expedition.

As Underhill observed, Sherman had assembled a large fleet of steamboats from St. Louis and Cairo, fifty-nine listed in his order, and Admiral Porter took his entire gunboat fleet from Memphis. The first troops embarked at Memphis on December 19th, and on December 21st, General Steele's crowded on at Helena. Among the transports were several that Underhill mentions: the *Forest Queen*, the general headquarters boat; the *J. W. Cheesman*, and the *Anglo-Saxon.* The Ohio 14th does not appear on Sherman's order, but the other regiments Underhill mentions were embarked as follows: the Ohio 16th on the *Henry von Phul;* the Ohio 42nd on the *Des Moines;* the Ohio 54th on the *Sunny South;* the Ohio 114th on the *Fanny Bullitt;* and the Ohio 120th on the *Northerner.* But they did not linger at Helena. As Underhill notes on December 23, "Before dark last night the last boat had left on its way down the river. Our division is the only one left here." Some 32,000 troops were headed south. In Helena, those left behind awaited news reports.

On December 27, he writes, "No news yet from the fleet that a few days since went down the river." But on New Year's Day 1863 he notes "Rumors of fighting at Vicksburg." On December 29, Sherman had launched an attack at Chickasaw Bayou just north of Vicksburg and had been forced to withdraw. In Vicksburg, news of the impending attack came during a holiday ball. A senior officer, calling for everyone's attention, halted the festivities and ordered the men to prepare for battle. Unfortunately for Sherman, Van Dorn had attacked Grant's supply depot at Holly Springs, cutting off his communications to Sherman and pulling him north, and Sherman's abortive assault in part resulted from Grant's inability to reach him.

Immediately after Sherman's defeat at Chickasaw Bayou, General John McClernand arrived on scene, and being senior to Sherman, took over his command. McClernand was determined to take Arkansas Post, and in a January 13, 1863 entry, Underhill's earlier musing whether "another attempt will be made to dislodge them" is answered, when he writes, "Gen. Gorman...brings reports of the capture of Arkansas Post." Forces under General McClernand, with assistance from Admiral Porter's gunboats, captured the post on January 11, although the 46th Indiana was not involved. Grant, who had no love for McClernand, was initially skeptical of the operation but later came to see that the move had been wise.

With the capture of Arkansas Post, operations in Arkansas ceased to be important, although after returning from the expedition down the Tallahatchie and Coldwater rivers, the Indiana 46th did go up the White River in January on an expedition under General Gorman. Underhill went on this expedition, and his entries from January 11-21, 1863 detail this.

On January 16, he writes: "The *Blue Wing* captured by the Secesh about the time of the late Vicksburg expedition is only a few hours ahead of us. *Rocket* has been dispatched after her but will probably not overtake her." A few days before the assault at Chickasaw Bayou, the *Blue Wing*, en route to the Yazoo from Memphis, towing coal barges and loaded with ammunition, had been hijacked by a Confederate boat that came out of the Arkansas River and took the *Blue Wing* upriver to Fort Hindman. The ammunition, destined for Sherman's use in the assault, was later found at the fort and reclaimed.

The 46th Indiana returned to Helena on January 23, 1863 and camped for their first morning ashore on the river bank. Later that day, they went into camp a mile back from the river. After three days of rain, the mud was terrible, as was Underhill's mood. Underhill rather acidly summarizes the expedition in his January 25 entry: "Result of expedition may thus be summed up: Cost about one million, a great deal wear and tear and accomplished the unnecessary feat of burning a number of out-houses at various places along the river."

Grant still wanted a way into Vicksburg from the rear. Sherman's assault at Chickasaw Bayou in December had failed. The canal across the peninsula to avoid the batteries along the river had failed. Work started the previous summer on the canal had recommenced on February 2, but on March 8, the rapidly rising river flooded the work, floating away tools and sending workers scampering for higher ground. While the canal work was going on, Grant had carried out some work on a plan to open up a water route through Louisiana via Lake Providence and several rivers, issuing into the Mississippi many miles below Vicksburg, but after that plan proved impractical, it was abandoned.

Now Grant concocted another scheme. He was eager to find a way into the Yazoo River above Haines Bluff, which had been too strongly fortified for the fleet to pass, and explains what he was trying to do:

> Lieutenant-Colonel Wilson of my staff was sent to Helena...to examine and open a way through Moon Lake and the Yazoo Pass if possible. Formerly there was a route by way of an inlet from the Mississippi river into Moon Lake, a mile east of the river, thence east through Yazoo Pass to Coldwater, along the latter to the Tallahatchie, which joins the Yallabusha about two hundred and fifty miles below Moon Lake and forms the Yazoo River. These were formerly navigated by steamers trading with the rich plantations along their banks, but the

> State of Mississippi had built a strong levee across the inlet some years before, leaving the only entrance for vessels into this rich region the one by way of the mouth of the Yazoo several hundred miles below.[16]

The Indiana 46th went on two expeditions involving the Yazoo Pass. The first one lasted about a week, and Underhill, left behind in camp near Helena, records on February 18, 1863 the beginning of the operation:

> Reg't left morning of 15th to assist in clearing Yazoo pass of obstructions – return perhaps first of next week. A channel is being opened up from Miss. River through a bayou to Moon Lake, thence through other bayous, into Coldwater which empties into the Talahatchie a tributary of the Yazoo. If opened up this channel will let us into the Yazoo in the rear of batteries placed on that river. The Rebels are busy blocking up the channel beyond where our men are at work. Many years since the channel was navigated particularly by flat boats. Navigation was closed by the levee being built....

The levee had been cut a few miles downstream of Helena on February 2, before the expedition left, causing much of the land east of it to flood and making dry ground to camp on hard to find. The regiment worked near Moon Lake, cutting trees and clearing timber. On February 19, Underhill reports, "Orders rec'd to prepare 15 days rations for another move. Regt not returned yet." It returned February 23, exhausted. But there was to be no rest for the weary. The regiment was in Helena for only a day before it was sent off again, this time for substantially longer.

On February 24, General Ross and 4500 men on fifteen transports, including the 46th, as well as two gunboats and a ram, left Helena on this Yazoo Pass expedition, and on February 25, Underhill notes, "Yesterday our entire division left down the Yazoo Pass. Perhaps be gone two or three weeks. Regt only returned day before leaving one man—Private George Bruington Co. B. – was wounded in Coldwater—wound received in calf of left leg." But progress was slow. The Confederates blocked the waterway with trees, and clearing all this took much time.

On March 4, the regiment was still away. "Yesterday returned from the Regt several sick men and this morning sent back about 30 convalescents under charge of Lt Andrew Co.A. Regt. when last heard from were in Coldwater River, having passed through Moon Lake."

Clearly the work there was rough, as we learn in his March 10 entry. "Regt still down the Yazoo Pass. Boats returning from there show they have been much damaged by their trip – chimneys knocked down, wheelhouses torn off rudders lost, and every conceivable injury rec'd from trees, and boughs of trees, snags too." One boat, the *Volunteer*, a very handsome new stern-wheeler fresh from Monongahela, became General Ross' flagship. By the end of the expedition, she reportedly looked like an old scow. Eventually, on March 11, General Ross arrived at the junction of the Tallahatchie and Yallabusha Rivers, where the Yazoo begins and where the Confederates had established Fort Pemberton, manned by five thousand men. Gunboats and troops attacked both on March 11 and 13 but failed to dislodge the enemy.

Because Fort Pemberton was only two feet above water, another cut was made in the Mississippi levee, this time directly across from Helena, with the hope that more water flooding in would wash away the fort. This effort was unsuccessful, however.

On March 21, Underhill was still at Helena and not destined to join his regiment:

> Early part of present week returned Dr Horace Coleman. Next morning started in company with all the Surgeons of Division remaining here to join the Division. Our division had proceeded as far as Greenwood at the mouth of the Tallahatchie River. There the Talla-

> hatchie and Yallabusha unite to form the Yazoo distant from here by water about 200 miles. Rebels have fortifications there and some fighting has been going on. News rec'd that Stewart of Co: B. was mortally wounded, Rogers of the same Co: severely wounded – Col. Bringhurst struck with piece of shell on the arm injured but little. But two surgeons Dr Varny and myself are left here in care of the sick of the division.

On March 26, the regiment was still away. "Day before yesterday returned from the Regt. Lieut. George W. Spencer came to take all men able for duty sent down 40 – old soldiers generally. Wright Nield, Private Co D- had his arm blown off by a cannon ball at Greenwood Miss. Arm afterwards amputated by Dr Dicken Brigade Surgeon and subject died in a few days." On March 31 Underhill writes, "Sick came up from the Pass. Report our regiment at Greenwood and fight imminent." On April 2, he heard that, "our division was on their route back from Greenwood – leaving Quimby's brigade there also some gunboats. Haines Bluff evacuated few days ago." Grant abandoned this route to get to Vicksburg after concluding he would have to get into the Yazoo River below the fort.

Grant's final winter attempt at Vicksburg came in March, after the Yazoo Pass attempt had failed. Admiral Porter took some gunboats a short distance up the Yazoo, then left the river, intending to navigate through various bayous until he could get back into the Yazoo below Fort Pemberton but above heavily fortified Haines Bluff, twelve miles from its mouth, and then come south towards Vicksburg. In one area, he literally had to cut his way through low overhanging trees, and because his progress was so slow, Confederates were able to attack him. The gunboats were useless in such a tight situation and Porter sent a desperate message to Sherman to rescue the expedition from the attackers. Sherman eventually did, but it then took several days to back the boats down and get them back to the mouth of the Yazoo.

By April 9, the Yazoo Pass expedition was over for the 46th, which was back at Helena. Underhill wrote,"Yesterday afternoon returned the regt. from Yazoo Pass Expedition. Since they left they have lost killed two wounded six and drowned one. Expedition a failure." And then he goes on rather ominously: "Rumored that we leave for Vicksburg to-morrow. Regt. still lying on boat."

Vicksburg

The rumors were true. The regiment never got off the *Volunteer*. General Hovey met the boat when it reached Helena and instructed the troops to remain aboard. On April 10, 1863, Underhill was embarked along with the 46th, and on the 11th the regiment left Helena for good, heading downriver as a part of McGinnis' Brigade of General Hovey's Division of the Thirteenth Army Corps, under the command of Major General McClernand.

Despite General Grant's unsuccessful attempts throughout the winter to take Vicksburg, his troops had been kept busy and hardened physically. Although Grant still considered moving his troops below Vicksburg by water, spring and warm weather had begun to dry out the land, making roads passable once again after a winter that had been unusually wet. Thus in April, Grant put a new plan into action.

He transported many of his troops to Milliken's Bend, Louisiana, today no longer there but then a community of about five hundred on the Mississippi shore about twenty-five miles above Vicksburg. Grant had concluded that the only way to get his troops into the rear of Vicksburg was to march them down the Louisiana side of the Mississippi and then transport them across the river at a point below the city. The 46th Indiana marched out of Milliken's Bend on April 16, and Underhill's entries from then until April 30, the day he crossed the river into Mississippi, describe that march.

In order to transport his troops across the river, Grant had to get both gunboats and transports below Vicksburg. This involved running a

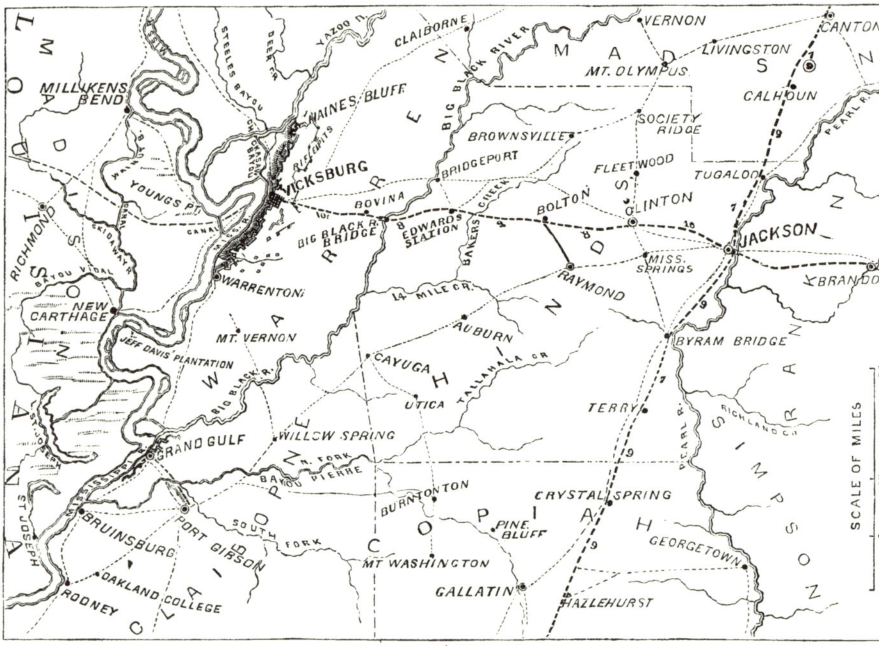

MAP ILLUSTRATING GRANT'S VICKSBURG CAMPAIGN.

A period map shows the scene of the Vicksburg Campaign in which Underhill took part. Union forces surged northeast towards Jackson, the Mississippi state capitol, then west close to the rail line. Between Bolton and Edwards Station, Underhill took part in the Battle of Champion Hill before heading west to Vicksburg, where his unit took part in the siege.

gauntlet of shore batteries that Grant estimated at fourteen miles. The vessels went in several groups, the gunboats protecting the transports, while the troops were marching overland. Grant tells of the first group:

> [On the 16th of April, the same day the 46th had left Milliken's Bend] the advance, flagship *Benton*, Porter commanding, started at ten o'clock at night, followed at intervals of a few minutes by the *Lafayette* with a captured steamer, the *Price*, lashed to her side, the *Louisville*, *Mound City*, *Pittsburgh*, and *Carondelet* – all

> those being naval vessels. Next came the transports – *Forest Queen*, *Silver Wave*, and *Henry Clay*, each towing barges loaded with coal to be used as fuel by the naval and transport steamers when below the batteries. The gunboat *Tuscumbia* brought up the rear. Soon after the start a battery between Vicksburg and Warrenton opened fire across the intervening peninsula, followed by the upper batteries, and then by batteries all along the line. The gunboats ran up close under the bluffs, delivering their fire in return at short distances, probably without much effect. They were under fire for more than two hours, and every vessel was struck many times, but with little damage to the gunboats. The transports did not fare so well. The *Henry Clay* was disabled and deserted by her crew. Soon after a shell burst in the cotton packed about the boilers, set the vessel on fire and burned her to the water's edge. The burning mass, however, floated down to Carthage [Louisiana] before grounding, as did also one of the barges in tow.[17]

Because of problems moving enough supplies overland, six more steamers, loaded with supplies and towing a dozen barges carrying rations, ran the batteries a few nights later, on the night of April 22. On April 24 Underhill wrote, "Night before last quite a number of transports ran the Rebel blockade and are now below Vicksburg. One or two were destroyed." On April 25 he noted, "The boats that ran the blockade the last night were the *Empire City*, *Moderator*, *Anglo-Saxon*, and *J. W. Cheeseman*. The *Tigress* in making the attempt was almost destroyed. The loss was 22 killed and wounded. The *Henry Clay* was not burned as reported a few nights ago in her attempt to run the blockade." But Underhill had his news wrong. We know from Grant that she was.

With some delays because of bayous needing bridging, Underhill and the 46th had marched to a point below Vicksburg on the Louisiana shore of the Mississippi, where they were then to embark on transports to take them across to a landing point south of Grand Gulf, Mississippi. Grand Gulf was fortified, and the gunboats were to put the guns there out of action before the transports would pass. Grant narrates:

> On the morning of the 29th [April 1863], McClernand was directed to embark all the troops from his corps that our transports and barges could carry. About 10,000 men were so embarked. The plan was to have the navy silence the guns at Grand Gulf, and to have as many men as possible ready to debark in the shortest possible time under cover of the fire of the navy and carry the works by storm.

Grant continues:

> At 8 o'clock AM., 29th, Porter made the attack with his entire strength present, eight gunboats. For nearly five and a half hours the attack was kept up without silencing a single gun of the enemy. All this time McClernand's 10,000 men were huddled together on the transports in the stream ready to attempt a landing if signalled.[18]

Underhill observed all this on April 29, near Grand Gulf, 11 AM:

> Yesterday we embarked on Forest Queen and came down arriving here before daylight this morning. We are nearly 4 miles distant lying on our transport watching the fight between the enemys batteries and our gunboats. The ball opened at 8 o'clock this morning and has continued with little intermission till present time. If the batteries are silenced we will land our troops from

> the transports. Four divisions are here Gens Grant, McPherson, McClernand – also Adjutant Gen Thomas and Gov. Yates of Illinois.

About 1:30 that afternoon, the fleet withdrew after it became evident that their fire was doing no good. Grant went aboard the navy flagship to confer. He and Admiral Porter arranged that for their safety, the troops would land above Grand Gulf and march across a peninsula on the Louisiana side to a point below, while the gunboats and transports ran the batteries. Porter agreed once they were below the batteries to use his gunboat fleet as well for transports. The 46th disembarked from the *Forest Queen* at Hard Times, Louisiana, and marched overland to DeShroon's plantation, below Grand Gulf but about six miles above Bruinsburg, Mississippi. Grant had anticipated landing at Rodney, further down, but he chose Bruinsburg after being informed that he would find a good landing area and a good road from there to Port Gibson.

On the morning of April 30, 1863, Underhill crossed the Mississippi on the flagship *Benton*, the Indiana 46th on the gun deck, the 24th on the upper deck, Admiral Porter and General Grant standing at the wheelhouse. As soon as the *Benton* reached the bank, both regiments disembarked, the first units to land.

Underhill writes in an evening entry on that day:

> This evening finds us camped a few miles below in the rear of Grand Gulf. Bombardment was kept up yesterday till 2 o'clock PM making a six hour fight. Of the 8 Rebel batteries two could not be silenced. Troops landed and marched across stinking river below. Transports ran by the batteries without material damage. Heavy bombardment little after dark. Entire loss on gunboats as follows: *Benton* 7 killed and 12 wounded – *Pittsburgh* 6 killed and 20 wounded – *Tuscumbia* 5 killed and 19 wounded – Some reported injured on the other boats. 7

> boats engaged – *Benton*, *Pittsburgh*, *Lafayette*, *Tuscumbia*, *Mound City*, *Louisville*, *Carondelet*. Our regt crossed this morning on *Benton*. 4 divisions on this side of river now.

Four divisions on the Mississippi side of the river represented a fraction of Grant's troops. Many had still to come across, leaving Grant vulnerable. Anticipating a landing below Vicksburg, General John Pemberton, commanding the forces at Vicksburg, had sent forces south. Had he concentrated all his forces south of Vicksburg, he might well have been able to stop Grant. But Grant had foreseen this. On April 29, the day before Grant landed at Bruinsburg, General Sherman led a feint against Haines Bluff, on the Yazoo, north of Vicksburg. On receiving the news of Sherman's deliberately open thrust, Pemberton turned his troops around and sent them north to ward off Sherman. As an additional distraction, Grant had ordered a cavalry raid under Colonel Benjamin Grierson that had left southern Tennessee on April 17, moving south in a destructive path through Mississippi, ending up at Baton Rouge on May 2nd. Thus, Grant succeeded in keeping Pemberton as close as possible to Vicksburg while he made his landing, as well as causing him to scatter his remaining forces in the north repelling Sherman and hunting for Grierson. This greatly reduced the threat Grant faced upon landing his troops, and the night of April 29, he sent word to Sherman to break off and join him immediately.

For the next six weeks, Grant was concerned with a relatively small theater that stretched from Jackson, Mississippi, the state capital, west about forty-five miles to Vicksburg, generally not far from the rail line that connected the two towns. Stops along the line east from Vicksburg included Edwards Station, Bolton Depot, Clinton, and finally Jackson. Raymond lies about half way between Bolton Depot and Clinton and about seven miles south. Underhill mentions all these in the diary.

From Bruinsburg, Union forces had to fight their way northeast. Grant's first fight was the Battle of Port Gibson on May 1, where

23,000 Union forces defeated 6000 Confederate forces under General Bowen. The 46th Indiana was involved. Underhill writes on Saturday morning, May 2nd:

> Day before yesterday marched from the river at 3 PM. Marched all night and arrived at the outposts of the enemy about daylight. 1st Ind. Battery lost one or two killed and 7 wounded. We took ½ hour's sleep and a little coffee. Carr's division moved on the enemy at 6 o'clock and our division (Gen Hovey's) came up just as they were beginning to give away at 7 o'clock a terrific fight occurred in which we finally drove the enemy from the field capturing a number of prisoners and two batteries of artillery. Our division was engaged about 8 hours and our brigade 5 hours. Loss of regt. and division impossible to ascertain as yet. The entire loss, however, is heavy. Rebels fought with the greatest desperation and bravery but we drove them at every point and are now only 2 ½ miles from Port Gibson. Last night we were called up but the alarm was false. Both parties have been reenforced during the last night and the contest may be renewed this morning unless the enemy fall back. Our regt and 24th Ind made the charge and took two batteries – the 46th taking as many prisoners as the regt. numbered.

Port Gibson 11 o'clock

> Enemy crossed bayou [Bayou Pierre] and in their retreat perhaps they will make a stand this side Black River. They burned the bridge behind them. We are now constructing bridges across the bayou to follow them. Port Gibson a nice town. When citizens at home number

> perhaps three thousand – county seat of Claiborne County. This morning on march found good many dead Secesh. Genl Tracy reported killed. Our regimental loss was 8 killed 36 wounded 4 to 6 of whom are mortally, many slightly wounded not reported. Distance from here to the point where we marched from on the Mississippi is 18 miles – 17 miles to the Black River 8 miles distant to Grand Gulf.

After the fight at Port Gibson, the 46th Indiana moved northeast but with a brief halt for rations and to allow troops in the rear to catch up. Grant wanted to move fast. He needed to take Jackson before it could be reinforced, since it was a major rail hub and if Confederate forces there could be defeated, they could not reinforce Pemberton to the west. After knocking out the threat at Jackson, he then would head west towards Vicksburg, having successfully separated Pemberton on the west from General Joseph Johnston's forces on the east.

In earlier operations, Grant had found that he could do without elaborate supply lines and move quickly, and in this operation the troops were traveling light. As Underhill had written on April 18 on the march from Milliken's Bend, "We camp without tents, our tents baggage etc. being left on transport Cheeseman. Slept under the stars last two nights." Grant intended to live off the land, something he had done successfully earlier. He writes:

> McClernand's and McPherson's commands were kept substantially as they were on the night of the 2nd, awaiting supplies sufficient to give them three days' rations in haversacks. Beef, mutton, poultry, and forage were found in abundance. Quite a quantity of bacon and molasses was also secured from the country, but bread and coffee could not be obtained in sufficient quantity for all the men....On the 6th...three days' rations had

> been brought up from Grand Gulf for the advanced troops and were issued. Orders were given for a forward movement the next day.[19]

Underhill notes all this. On May 4 he writes, " Moved camp about one mile rested during day – boys were out foraging great portion of the time. Weather warm and dry. Grand Gulf was taken possession of yesterday." On the 5th, he writes, "Remained here all day waiting for rations – not yet come." On the 7th, he comments on rations: "Yesterday morning took up line of march at 5 o'clock, made 8 miles by 9 o'clock and went into camp. Here we will probably remain till we get rations. Provision is getting scarce and we are compelled to forage."

Grant was pleased with what was happening, according to Underhill's May 8 entry:

> Have not changed camp to day. Forces reviewed by Maj. Gen. Grant – an order read from him complimenting the army on their achievements – amongst the rest gave the number of prisoners captured near Port Gibson at one thousand. Promised the principal part of our hardships would soon be over but said that more battles were first to be fought.

The 46th continued moving northeast, still traveling light, as Underhill notes on May 9:

> Since we left Milliken's Bend have not been sheltered by tents. Arrange a few green boughs to form a shade beneath which we lie lazily during the heat of the day. The same arrangement also suffices to intercept the heavy dews that fall. Make our beds on the ground and sleep with lizards and snakes with which country abounds.

On May 10, the 46th marched through Cayuga. On the 12th, after some skirmishing, they camped at Baker's Creek, about four miles northeast of Raymond and roughly half way between Raymond and Clinton. On the 13th and 14th, the 46th moved in the area around Raymond, and Underhill recorded the Battle of Raymond on the 12th, although the 46th Indiana was not involved. Sherman and McPherson's forces headed for Jackson, where they attacked 6,000 Confederates and on May 14, the Confederates withdrew.

On May 15 at Bolton Depot, Underhill writes:

> News rec'd this morning of the capture of Jackson the Capital by Gen. McPherson's corps. Our division moved to Clinton distant 4 miles thence to this station on the Vicksburg & Jackson Rail Road. Making a march of 12 miles. Arrived here about noon and will probably remain to-night. Clinton on the main rail road route a town numbering about 600 – quite a number citizens there – saw many of the "fair Secesh." We are now between Jackson and Vicksburg distant from the former 15 miles and the latter 40. Campaign so far has been successful beyond my most sanguine expectations.

Jackson having been taken and General Johnston's forces having retreated north to Canton, Grant then wanted to move west essentially along the railroad towards Vicksburg. This, however, was not without incident. On the night of May 14, he received an intercepted message from General Johnston to General Pemberton. Johnston wanted Pemberton to come east to Grant's rear at Clinton. Grant was fearful lest Johnston cut north of him and over towards Vicksburg to join up with Pemberton. Sherman and McPherson had been left in Jackson to destroy its rail and military manufacturing facilities, but Grant ordered them to Bolton at once. On May 16, Hovey's division of McClernand's corps, which included the 46th Indiana, was the first to engage Pemberton's forces at Champion Hill, named after the family which owned, and still owns, the land several miles east of Edwards Station where the battle was fought. A nasty battle ensued that lasted some four hours but which was preceded by skirmishing which essentially amounted to battle. Because of a gap which developed in the line, many of Pemberton's forces were able to retreat. Grant was singularly displeased with General McClernand, feeling that had he moved up when ordered, Pemberton would never have escaped. On Saturday night, May 16, Underhill describes the battle, his entry made too early yet to call it the Battle of Champion Hill:

> Reveille at half past three o clock this morning. Took up march little after daylight marched westward along a road parallel with the rail road from 5 to 8 miles till we came unexpectedly upon the pickets of the enemy. After reconnoitering as usual we finally made the attack with our division and after a hard fight succeeded in driving the enemy one and an half miles and taking six pieces of Artillery. The enemy however, being largely reenforced numbering three lines our division after a most desperate struggle drove us back over the whole of the ground we had taken but we being reenforced by Quinby's division again drove them back in return and held the field. Our division was under fire 6 ½ hours and lost heavily. Our Regt having perhaps the smallest loss and losing about 75 in killed and wounded. Some are also missing. Quinby's division lost heavily as also did Carr's which were all the troops engaged save a little sparring by General Logan. We are camped to night on the Rebel side of the battle-field. The loss of the enemy in killed and wounded is perhaps fully as great as our own although they had much the advantage in position. Besides their loss in prisoners was very heavy.

That Saturday night, the 46th was camped at the battlefield, and Sunday and Monday were grim clean-up days. Underhill tells us about Sunday:

> Been busy all day and last night in attentions to wounded – wrapped in my blanket and slept one hour last night among the bushes beneath the stars. Entire loss of our division in the battle of yesterday ascertained to be 1,306. Balance of troops save our brigade has gone in pursuit of enemy in direction of Black River. Our brigade remains to bury the dead. Not known when we will follow.

On Tuesday evening, May 19th, he reported that

> Yesterday our division was engaged in burying dead, collecting spoils of battle, and this day at noon we took up our line of march and are now on the north bank of Black River, bivouacked for the night – marched 10 miles this afternoon 15 yet to Vicksburg. Dr. Washburn left with our wounded near the battlefield – country through which we moved barren and desolate – more level, however, than further down. A sharp fight occurred to our advance at Black River. Since we have landed on this side of Mississippi have taken in all 7,000 prisoners besides their wounded and captured 90 pieces of artillery.

The Big Black River lies about eleven miles east of Vicksburg, and another battle had erupted there on May 17. Union forces pushed back the Confederates, who then retreated into Vicksburg. Grant pushed ahead and on May 19 launched an assault. This time, however, the Confederates were well protected behind fortifications, and they simply cut down the Union troops advancing over open ground.

By Thursday, May 21, the 46th was close to Vicksburg and traveling light was showing its disadvantages. Underhill writes:

> This evening finds us in camp just back of Vicksburg perhaps 3 miles distant from the city. Last night we commenced our march about dark and marched till midnight when we turned in an old field to rest till morning. I had no blanket so I had an uncomfortable time trying to sleep in the open air with nothing between myself and the ground and no covering of any kind whatever. Latter part of the nights are here at this season of the year decidedly cool no matter how warm may have been the previous day. Took up line of march this morning about sunrise and reached present encampment about 2 o'clock PM. About noon it rained heavily and most of us were completely soaked. We are now lying in a ravine behind the division of Osterhaus who is in the advance of this corps. Our corps – McClernand's occupies the left – McPherson's the center and Sherman's the right resting on the Yazoo. Haines Bluff has been evacuated. We are plying our Artillery on the enemy and have our sharpshooters so close upon them that they can scarcely get an opportunity to reply.

On May 22, Grant launched another massive assault on Vicksburg. This was preceded by an artillery bombardment both by naval forces on the river and land forces in the rear of the city. However, after this assault failed, as had his earlier one on May 19, Grant concluded that the only way he could take the city was to lay siege to it:

Underhill noted on May 25th,

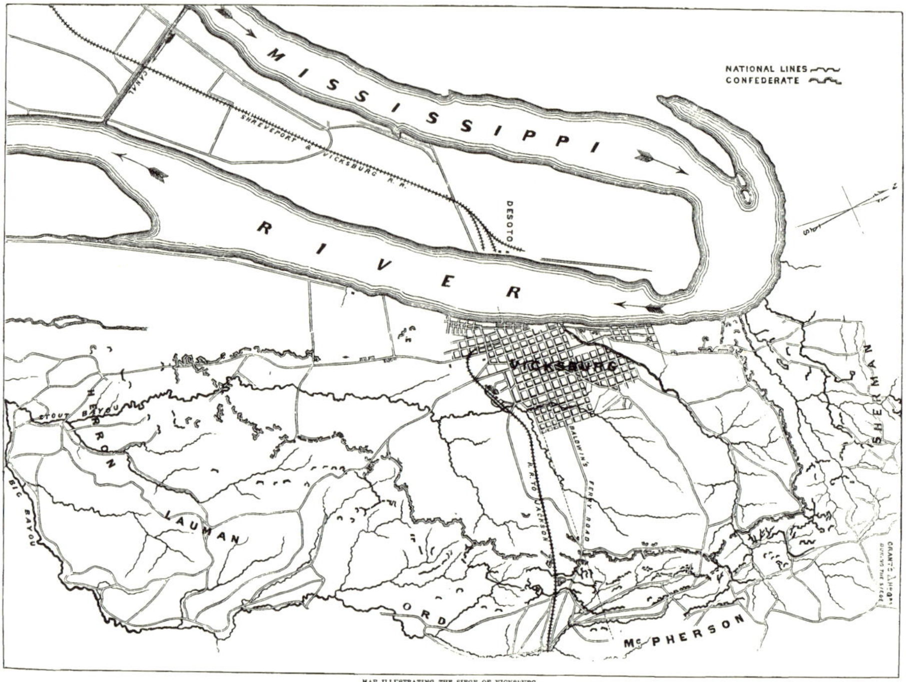

MAP ILLUSTRATING THE SIEGE OF VICKSBURG.

A detailed map of Vicksburg shows how close Confederate and Union lines were encamped to one another during the siege of the city. Underhill's Indiana regiment was in the Thirteenth Corps, intially commanded by General John A. McClernand, who was replaced during the siege by General Edward O. C. Ord.

Since last paragraph was written we have been lying in a ravine 400 yards distant from enemy's fortifications sharpshooting. Bullets fell around us quite plentifully – but none of our reg't hurt, however. Relieved this morning by 2nd Brigade. Pretty heavy fighting on the 22nd inst. Seems determined that we will take place of Vicksburg by regular siege rather than direct attack. Reenforced by Hurlbuts corps. From the point where our sharpshooters were stationed we could distinctly hear at night the barking of dogs in the city – the town clock

> striking – carriages rattling over the streets and such like sounds. Flag of truce came over from the Rebels about 2 o'clock this afternoon for the purpose of burying their dead. We also occupied the time in burying our dead who had fallen near the enemy's works. The occasion of respite was enjoyed hugely by both parties. Boys were close enough together to carry on ordinary conversation. In fact some of ours as well as theirs crossed the lines and becoming mixed were obliged to be sent back by their respective commanders. This evening returned Chaplain Robb from the Hospital where our wounded at "Champion Hill" were left. Reports that Lt. Andrews and Private Butler are dead – balance doing well. Have not yet been captured by Guirrellas although in the enemy's country. Goes back to-morrow or next day.

On Friday, May 29, the city-class gunboat *Cincinnati* was hit by guns at Vicksburg, and sank. The Southerners exulted. Only in August, after the siege, was she raised and towed to Cairo. Underhill's entry for that day is brief: "This morning for half an hour from 6 till 6 ½ and this evening from half past 5 o'clock till six a most terrific bombardment took place – without, however, much apparent effect. One house only known to be burned." Mrs. Emma Balfour, a resident of Vicksburg, kept a diary during the siege. Her entry for May 30 is considerably longer and suggests that there was much more effect than Underhill noted. Part of her entry reports:

> ...the most fearful cannonading commenced from the lines. I never saw anything like it. The shells fell *literally* like hail. Mrs. Willis' house was struck twice and two horses in front of her door were killed. It only lasted an hour and a great deal of damage was done in that time. Three persons in town were killed, all servants....I hear

> this morning that a bomb exploded in the court house, killing two men and wounding seven, and in another house several were injured. I could hear the pieces falling all around us as the shell would explode, and once I thought our time had come.... They [the mortar shells] come gradually making their way higher and higher, tracked by their firing fuse till they reach their greatest altitude – then with a rush and whiz they come down furiously, their own weight added to the impetus given by the powder. Then look out, for if they explode before reaching the ground which they generally do, the pieces fly in all directions – the very least of which will kill one and most of them of sufficient weight to tear through a house from top to bottom.[20]

As the siege progresses, Underhill's diary entries grow much shorter, since the men simply had to wait for a surrender. On June 19, however, he makes an interesting comment rather at variance with common opinion in the higher command echelons. He writes,

> Gen. McClernand commanding our corps is to be relieved by Major Gen. Ord. Probable cause personal difficulty with Gen. Grant. To be regretted – McClernand is one of our most successful generals second only in military ability to Gen. Grant in this Department and probably not to him.

In both General Grant's and General Sherman's memoirs and elsewhere, a different picture emerges. John A. McClernand was an Illinois Democrat who had served in the U.S. House of Representatives from 1843-1851 and from 1859-1861. He had left the House to seek a military command. He was an arrogant, self-promoting, egotistical man who derided West Point graduates and mocked their caution. He was, however, a staunch supporter of the war whose support Lincoln needed. In mid 1862, McClernand inveigled Lincoln and Secretary of War Stanton into letting him raise and command his own force which would operate independently within Grant's theater of command. He would act boldly and asserted he could take Vicksburg by Christmas. This was done quietly as a private deal between them – Grant was not informed – but as time went on, General Henry Halleck, Army Commander in Chief, who had had no fondness for Grant, recognized that whatever drawbacks he might have, Grant was a proven soldier with sound training, whereas McClernand, of whom he did not approve, was something of a loose cannon. Gradually what had happened reached Grant, who asked that the lines of authority be made clear to him. To McClernand's chagrin, Halleck authorized sending the troops McClernand had recruited to Grant's command, where Grant was senior. Like Halleck, Grant had no confidence in McClernand as a military leader, and although the trouble with McClernand had started earlier, it erupted during the planning for the January expedition against Arkansas Post immediately after McClernand had relieved Sherman following the Chickasaw Bayou debacle.

After the *Blue Wing* had been hijacked about December 20, 1862 by a Confederate boat and taken to Fort Hindman at Arkansas Post, Sherman and Admiral Porter had discussed the issue and concluded that the post should be taken lest further incidents occur. On the night of January 4 [Porter says it was December 31], Sherman took McClernand aboard the flagship late at night to discuss the matter with Porter, who had been most cooperative with Sherman and Grant. On this occasion, McClernand made a cutting remark about Sherman's recent defeat, which angered Porter. Sherman writes:

> We were seated in [Porter's]cabin and I explained my views about Arkansas Post and asked his cooperation....Porter's manner to McClernand was so curt that I invited him out into a forward-cabin where he had his

> charts, and asked him what he meant by it. He said that "he did not like him;" that in Washington, before coming West, he had been introduced to him by President Lincoln, and he had taken a strong prejudice against him. I begged him, for the sake of harmony, to waive that, which he promised to do.[21]

In an extract from his journal which he sent to Sherman in 1875, Porter notes indignantly that McClernand suggested moving against Arkansas Post as if it had been his own idea. Porter deeply resented McClernand's treating Sherman rudely.

McClernand had arrived second in command to Grant. Grant writes:

> ...[After the Arkansas Post expedition] I received messages from both Sherman and Admiral Porter, urging me to come and take command in person, and expressing their distrust of McClernand's ability and fitness for so important and intricate an expedition [against Vicksburg].
>
> On the 17 I visited McClernand and his command at Napoleon. It was here made evident to me that both the army and the navy were so distrustful of McClernand's fitness to command that, while they would do all they could to insure success, this distrust was an element of weakness. It would have been criminal to send troops under these circumstances into such danger. By this time I had received authority to relieve McClernand, or to assign any person else to the command of the river expedition, or to assume command in person. I felt great embarrassment about McClernand. He was the senior major-general after myself within the department. It would not do, with his rank and ambition, to assign a junior over him. Nothing was left but to assume the

> command myself. I would have been glad to put Sherman in command, to give him an opportunity to accomplish what he had failed in the December before; but there seemed no other way out of the difficulty, for he was junior to McClernand. Sherman's failure needs no apology.[22]

Sherman later reports that

> McClernand's report of the capture of Fort Hindman [at Arkansas Post] almost ignored the action of Porter's fleet altogether. This was unfair, for I know that the admiral led his fleet in person in the river-attack, and that his guns silenced those of Fort Hindman, and drove the gunners into the ditch.[23]

In several references, Grant is critical of McClernand. He blamed McClernand for the escape of Pemberton's forces at Champion Hill, and in the assault on Vicksburg on May 22, Grant felt that McClernand had misrepresented his successes and unnecessarily asked for reinforcements. Grant's firing of McClernand is terse:

> On the 17th [of June] I received a letter from General Sherman and one on the 18th from General McPherson saying that their respective commands had complained to them of a fulsome, congratulatory order published by General McClernand to the 13th corps, which did great injustice to the other troops engaged in the campaign...I at once wrote to McClernand, directing him to send me a copy of this order. He did so, and I at once relieved him from command of the 13th army corps and ordered him back to Springfield, Illinois. The publication of his order in the press was in violation of War Department orders and also of mine.[24]

One can only surmise that Grant had been waiting for his chance to sack McClernand.

The siege had not let up since it began May 22. On June 20th, Underhill writes:

> This A.M. at 4 o'clock all the land artillery nearly 200 pieces in number – the gunboats and mortar fleet opened up on the city – and rained a terrible fire for six hours – Not much visible effect.

A private with the 20th Ohio Infantry Regiment reported that the firing along the seven mile front created so much smoke that no one could see anything.

As the siege progressed, conditions in Vicksburg became desperate. The constant fire, both from the rear and from the river, wrecked buildings and sent inhabitants into caves dug into the hills. Food became scarce. Beef became unavailable and people turned to mule meat. Commodity prices soared, flour reaching $1000 per barrel and meal $140 per bushel. The privations that people endured had by early July become so unbearable that on July 3, General Pemberton sent emissaries to Grant to work out a surrender.

Underhill writes on July 3:

> Siege still continues. This is the 46th day but from circumstances developed within the last few hours the place will probably be surrendered within the next 12 hours. This morning between the hours of 7 and 8 o'clock a flag of truce was sent by Gen. Pemberton to Gen. Grant asking that commissioners be appointed to fix the terms of surrender. Grant replied that it was unnecessary, as the surrender must be unconditional. Other dispatches have since been passing between the respective commanders but the result and purport have

> not been made known. Hostilities by the land force has been suspended since the flag of truce this morning except about an hour this afternoon by some misunderstanding our artillery and sharpshooters again opened out again. The Mortar fleet, however, not being informed of what was transpiring continued to throw their shells in every direction. They have certainly produced much havoc amongst the garrison. I saw one piece strike an angle of a fort – and in another case I saw a man wounded while I was watching within a period of half an hour. Of course, however, I could see but very little of the damage done by the mortars.

That afternoon, Grant and Pemberton met and eventually settled on the terms of surrender. The next day, July 4, 1863, Union forces took control of Vicksburg.

On July 4th, Underhill conveys the joy of the surrender:

> At 5 o'clock this morning all our large guns opened up and fired 35 rounds blank cartridges in honor of the glorious 4th. At precisely half past seven the City of Vicksburg surrendered. When the white flags were placed upon the forts in token of surrender enthusiastic shouts went up from thousands of our brave boys. The shouts were taken up and carried along the line for miles. Number of prisoners twenty two thousand 15,000 effective and 7,000 unfit for duty – largest capture ever made on the American Continent...

For the Union, that Independence Day was a glorious one, for also on that day, Union forces won the battle at Gettysburg. But for the inhabitants of Vicksburg, the defeat was so devastating that not until 1945 would citizens there once again celebrate the Fourth of July.

Feelings were mixed. When there was minor looting by Federal troops, Grant put an immediate stop to it. He kept the prisoners in their own camps, under their old commanders. The Union troops seemed to feel mostly a deep sympathy for what the Confederates had suffered. There appeared to be no jeering or gloating. Union troops shared their relatively bountiful provisions with the starving Confederates.

Underhill's unit, however, received orders to move off immediately after the surrender. In another entry on July 4, we sense his pique: "We are vexed... and it takes half the pleasure of the capture that our division move away this evening without even getting a sight of the city. Late this evening I was down in the suburbs of the city and examined the Rebel works." But Grant's rear was being threatened, and he put Sherman in command of the troops having to deal with it.

During the whole time that Pemberton had been holed up in Vicksburg with an estimated 30,000 men, the Confederates had been hoping that General Joe Johnston would come to attack Grant from the rear. Johnston felt his force was too weak, and no reinforcements were available. Johnston had thought Pemberton should break out in order to help him, but Pemberton was adamant that he was to hold on to Vicksburg and would not send out troops. Before Grant had swung west to Vicksburg, McPherson and Sherman had routed Johnston's forces from Jackson. The Confederates then fled north to Canton, whereupon Grant headed for Vicksburg. But it was feared that Johnston was amassing a force of 30,000 to 40,000 men at the Big Black River to attack Federal troops from the rear to allow Pemberton to escape. To prevent an attack, Grant had ordered Sherman to protect him. Therefore, from June 20 until July 4, Sherman had spread his forces out from Haines Bluff on the Yazoo over to the railroad bridge at Big Black. Underhill makes reference to this threat on July 1:

> Intelligence has been rec'd that the Rebel Gen. Bragg is reenforcing Johnson at Canton to attack our rear. Two divisions are reported as having already arrived there

> and the greatest part of Bragg's Army following. Yesterday a council of war was held – but the deliberations were of course not made known.

Immediately following the surrender at Vicksburg, orders were given to attack General Johnston. The 13th Corps, now under General Ord, following General McClernand's dismissal, was ordered to cross the Big Black River at the railroad bridge and to head for Bolton. The 46th Indiana headed out. Underhill tracks the progress. On Sunday July 5, he writes:

> Did not march at 5 o'clock yesterday evening – moved at 5 this morning had a hot dusty day's march. Made about 11 miles and stopped about two miles from Black River. Our whole corps is on the march. Was very sick to-day compelled to stop a few hours on the march and rest in the shade. Heavy cannonading heard this afternoon in a northwesterly direction.

On Monday, at 10 PM, he notes:

> Been lying under the shade of the oak trees resting all day. March again at 4 o'clock. As the result of fighting heard in the northwest yesterday a large number of prisoners were taken back towards Vicksburg – also an immense number of arms etc. Evidently the campaign is not yet over in the southwest. Day very hot.

That Monday the 46th had marched in late afternoon to the Big Black River bridge, where they camped for the night. Underhill made his bed of two cotton bales. On Tuesday, they crossed the river and

> ...marched 16 miles along the Mississippi & Jackson

> RR to Bolton Depot. Passed over the Battlefield "Champion Hill" which called up many sad memories. The enemy in considerable force under Breckenridge kept ahead of us – occasionally skirmishing a little with his rear. Rained very hard last night and got very wet and could not sleep. No protection from the storm which wet me to the skin making me in a bad humor all day. Of our corps Osterhaus is first in line 2nd Carr – 3rd Smith and 4th Hovey and 5th Lauman – making 5 divisions of the corps – small divisions however. We move again at 5 P.M.,. to day with 2 days rations and without teams.

By this time, Johnston had heard of Vicksburg's surrender and retreated fast to Jackson. The weather was extremely hot and water scarce. Writing on Friday, July 10, two miles west of Jackson, Underhill was indignant:

> Left Clinton this morning – at 8 o'clock arrived here before noon – enemy posted and entrenched in the city and surroundings. Water is difficult of access as all the ponds and cisterns have been rendered unfit for use by the Rebels killing hogs, cattle, mules, etc. and throwing them in the water – a detestable mode of warfare – unfit for civilized nations. Enemy appears pretty formidable. Composed probably of the forces under Johnson reenforced by Bragg. It is known that Breckenridge is there forces number perhaps fifty thousand pretty well entrenched. Ours will number as much besides the cavalry and artillery. Gen. Sherman is in command – Grant having remained at Vicksburg. The different corps of our army have taken several parallel roads till they arrived near Clinton where they converged. Weather hot – will camp to-night in a heavy wood south of the main road.

On July 14, Underhill writes of hearing the day before about the victory at Gettysburg, and while he does not refer to it, another Union victory had occurred on July 9. Simultaneous with the assault on Vicksburg, General Banks had tried to take Port Hudson, Louisiana, the other remaining Confederate stronghold on the Mississippi. Two assaults had proven fruitless, but with help from Admiral Farragut, he laid siege to the town. When its commander learned that Vicksburg had fallen and that Johnston was not coming to help, he surrendered, thus giving the Union at last one of its strategic objectives – full control of the Mississippi River.

General Johnston had hoped that Sherman would make a frontal assault on Jackson, but instead, Sherman deployed his forces around it in a semicircle, from the Pearl River north of the city around it to the Pearl on the south. In the attack on Jackson, General Lauman pressed forward too far too fast, with terrible losses. On July 14, Underhill recorded the event:

> Yesterday A.M. about 9 o'clock we again advanced cautiously heavy skirmishing all the time – pushed our division to within 1½ miles of the State Capitol our skirmishers having good view of the Rebel works. Our reg't was in the advance lost 8 men wounded – 4 supposed mortally – 11th Ind lost 7 wounded – entire division only about 33. Gen. Lauman's division coming in on our right was more unfortunate. It is said he disobeyed orders and in trying to advance too far was repulsed with severe loss – was immediately relieved of his command which has been temporarily given to our Gen. Hovey. He now commands 5 brigades.

And the next day Underhill noted that "Gen. Lauman's division lost 478 – in killed, wounded, and missing on the 13th Inst."

Sherman's account of the same event is rather poignant:

> On the 11th we pressed close in, and shelled the town from every direction. One of Ord's brigades (Lauman's) got too close, and was very roughly handled and driven back in disorder. General Ord accused the commander (General Lauman) of having disregarded his orders, and attributed to him personally the disaster and heavy loss of men. He requested his relief, which I granted, and General Lauman went to the rear, and never regained his division. He died after the war, in Iowa, much respected, as before that time he had been universally esteemed a most gallant and excellent officer.[25]

Sherman's forces shelled Jackson from 11-17 July, until they learned that the Confederates had evacuated. Underhill observes on July 17th:

> Jackson is evacuated – evacuated last night. Rode over town and fortifications – works were strong enough in themselves but our fire would pass over the first line and annoy the enemy at the opposite side. Might have been flanked. Enemy numbered forty thousand effective men. Town is almost entirely deserted very few families remaining – a desolate place. Boys are pillaging unmercifully – Burning many buildings not only public but private dwellings – Should not be permitted. War, civilized war, is bad enough, it should not be perverted from its original design. Ordered to hold ourselves in readiness to move at a moment's notice – probably return to the Mississippi River in the morning. Rail Road across the Pearl will be destroyed completely. Topography of the country a low plain covered with forest principally dwarf-oak – get water from artificial ponds generally except where we are camped we have access to creek.

On July 21, Underhill's prediction of returning to the Mississippi River proved correct. Reveille sounded at 2 AM and the regiment marched fourteen miles to camp that night in Raymond. July 21 would be the last entry in his diary during the war. Underhill years later explains why:

> I with some other soldiers had slept that night at a deserted farmhouse on our line of march. Early in the morning we hastily resumed our march and it was not for some hours subsequent that I discovered I had left my diary at the house already mentioned.

And thus Underhill's own account of his exploits with the 46th Indiana ended. The regimental history and other sources fill in what happened to the 46th after that time. Underhill's chagrin on July 4 at having to leave Vicksburg before he could see the city must in part have been mitigated, however, because after a needlessly punishing march from Jackson, the regiment reached Vicksburg on July 23. There it remained until August 4.

After Vicksburg

After the victory at Vicksburg on July 4, 1863 and the fall of Port Hudson on the 9th, the Mississippi River was once again under Union control. Both Generals Grant and Banks wanted to move immediately against Mobile, Alabama to prevent Confederate reinforcements for General Johnston from moving north, but international considerations led the Lincoln administration to overrule domestic ones. The French still wanted an empire in the New World, and in June 1863, French Army forces had overthrown the Mexican government. This was seen as a breach of the Monroe Doctrine. Lincoln refused to recognize the new government and recalled his envoy. The Confederacy, however, did offer to recognize it. Throughout the war, the Confederacy had been trying to gain diplomatic recognition both from England and France, but neither would act unilaterally. By recognizing the new government in Mexico, the Confederates hoped they would enhance their chances of gaining recognition by France and ultimately by Britain. When Confederates in Texas began cultivating Mexican opponents of the overthrown government, Lincoln felt the need to establish a Union presence in Texas to counter any threat, and in the summer of 1863, General Nathaniel Banks, Commander of the Department of the Gulf, was given instructions to occupy a point of his own choosing in Texas. Banks began planning to move against Houston by way of the Sabine Pass, and at this time, Grant sent the 13th Corps, to which the 46th Indiana belonged, to the Department of the Gulf.

The 46th, which had marched back to the Mississippi after the attack on Jackson, reached Vicksburg on July 23, utterly exhausted, and went into camp along the river just below the city. It paused there until August 4, when it shipped out aboard the side-wheel *Baltic* for Natchez, Mississippi, where it remained until August 15. During the time the 46th was at Natchez, and where he had another malaria attack, Underhill had a conflict with his colleague, Israel B. Washburn, which may have begun some time earlier. Horace Coleman, the first Surgeon of the regiment, had sent a letter on December 14, 1862 to Indiana Governor Morton, noting that the two assistant surgeons in the regiment, Dr. William Haymond and Dr. William Spencer, were resigning and recommended that Underhill and Washburn be promoted to take their places. He noted that

> Underhill is Hospital Steward but has been in reality Assistant Surgeon of the Regt. & proved himself industrious, capable, and honest. Dr. Washburn has served as Hospital Ward Master when with the regiment; having been detailed much of the time by Medical Directors as surgeon on special duty.

The commanding officer, Colonel Thomas H. Bringhurst, also recommended both, noting that "these gentlemen are regularly graduated practicing physicians...." Endorsing the recommendation were Doctors Jessup, Casselberry, Ellis, Dicken, and Horace Coleman. Governor Morton accepted the recommendation and commissioned both, Washburn's dating from 26 December 1862 and Underhill's from 30 December 1862.

On July 31, 1863, Dr. Coleman resigned. Underhill and Washburn, both Assistant Surgeons, wanted his job. For understandable reasons, Bringhurst did not want to decide this. In a letter to Governor Morton dated August 10, written at Natchez, with a number of recommended promotions, Bringhurst noted that his recommendations were made in accordance with a general order of the governor, all in the direct line of promotion. Then he got to Washburn and Underhill:

> The resignation of Horace Coleman, Surgeon, leaves a vacancy. The General Order referred to above deprives the regiment of one 1st Assistant Surgeon. We can, therefore, but promote one of our Assistants.
>
> Dr. Israel Washburn is the senior by commission and expects promotion under your General Order upon the subject. He presents testimonials of qualification.
>
> Dr. J. W. Underhill claims to be senior in being appointed to fill the vacancy occasioned by the resignation of Dr. Haymond, who was the senior Assistant Surgeon.
>
> I recommend that one of the Assistants above, be appointed Surgeon.

On the same day, Underhill himself wrote a letter directly to Governor Morton:

> As there may be some difficulty in determining which of the Assistant Surgeons are entitled to fill the position made vacant by the resignation of Surgeon Horace Coleman, I beg leave to submit the following:
>
> Although Dr. Washburn's commission is three days older than mine it was the intention of those who recommended both of us that I should be the Senior Assistant. Dr. Washburn was also satisfied that I should have the precedence and there must have been a mistake in the commission.
>
> I have been in the Regiment since its organization, have performed at least as much duty as any other member of the Medical Department and have – whenever Dr. Coleman was absent – been left in charge of the

> Regiment. When his resignation was accepted he transferred all Medical and Hospital property to me and left me in charge.
>
> The Medical Director decided that I was really the Senior Assistant since I was commissioned to fill the vacancy caused by Dr. Haymond's resignation – Dr. Haymond being the original Assistant Surgeon who came into the field with the Regiment while Dr. Washburn follows Spencer who had been appointed 2nd Ass't.
>
> I refer you to any of the field officers of our Regiment.

On October 19, 1863, from camp near Grand Coteau, Louisiana, Washburn also wrote directly to Governor Morton:

> On or about the 11th day of August last I forwarded recommendations for the appointment of Surgeon of the 46th Regt. Ind Vols. The recommendations were signed by Surgeon R. B. Jessup 24th Ind Vols and "Surgeon in Chief" 3rd Division 13th a.c.[Army Corps] J. A. Comington, Surgeon 11th Ind Vols and "Senior Surgeon 1st Brigade 3d Div. and J. L. Dicken Surgeon 41st Ind Vols and "Senior Surgeon" 2nd Brigade 3d Division.
>
> I am the Senior Assistant Surgeon of the 46th Regiment Ind Vols and a graduate of Rush Med College Chicago Ill. My colleague J. W.Underhill who is also an applicant for the same position is the junior Ass't Surgeon and is not a graduate of any of any [sic] school. I submit the above facts for your careful consideration....

Underhill on the initial muster roll had followed his name with M.D., and although his medical school record shows his degree date as 1865, he had effectively completed the degree requirements, even if officially he had not been granted the degree. Because Washburn had known Underhill well for some time and knew Underhill's background, his assertion that Underhill was not a medical school graduate is at best equivocation. We shall never know if Underhill was aware of Washburn's letter.

Governor Morton appears to have decided by pure seniority, and Washburn was commissioned Surgeon October 17th. However, shortly before his own resignation, Washburn did write Underhill a warm recommendation for promotion to Surgeon, as did Colonel Bringhurst, who added, "Dr. Underhill, I am glad to be able to say, possesses none of the vices that so frequently disgrace the service in the form of many of its officers."

On August 15, the 46th embarked on the side-wheel *Des Arc,* where they encountered some of the former officers from the *Golden State* who recalled the men from February 1862. They headed south, landing five miles above New Orleans at Carrollton on the 17th, where they remained for the next several weeks.

In early September 1863, Banks sent an expedition to gain control of the Sabine Pass, a passage between the Gulf of Mexico and Sabine Lake, into which the Sabine River, which forms the border between Louisiana and Texas, flows. Their immediate objective was Sabine City, at the top of the pass on the west side. The expedition was a disaster, and on the 11th, the forces returned to New Orleans. Following this, Banks considered two moves: the first, a move overland by way of Shreveport, in northwestern Louisiana, and the second, a move across southern Louisiana to the Sabine. He quickly moved troops to the Bayou Teche area in southwestern Louisiana, including the 46th Indiana, which left New Orleans September 12. Between then and December 19, when it returned to Algiers, just across the river from New Orleans, the regiment was operating in an area between Berwick and Opelousas, getting into an occasional skirmish and into a more serious fight near Grand Coteau. Underhill, however, participated in only part of this, since the regimental muster shows him detached for November and December in charge of the hospital at New Iberia, Louisiana.

He was, however, listed as present during the first four months of 1864. On January 2, the regiment reenlisted as veterans. It remained at Algiers until January 19, when it was taken across Lake Ponchartrain to Madisonville, where it remained in camp until February 27. On that date it returned to Algiers, and on March 4, it moved with General Banks' army on the Red River expedition whose objective was Shreveport, in northwestern Louisiana, on the Red River.

In undertaking this, Banks had made several conditions: that the expedition not go forward until the Red River had enough water for the naval vessels and heavy-draft transports; that there be enough forces; that it have time enough to defeat General Kirby Smith's forces; that the Vicksburg-Shreveport railroad be repaired so that a land supply line could be established; and that all operations be under the command of one general.

In the end, the campaign was a disaster. First, given other Union exigencies, almost no other forces were available, and ones loaned by Sherman were available for only a month. The month allotted would not have been sufficient to rebuild the rail line, and the expedition had to be completed before the drop in the river level during the summer. As well, putting all the forces under the command of one general was never carried out. Given that nothing of great strategic value was at stake, Banks should have abandoned the expedition, but he did not.

Admiral Porter had assembled a fleet of fifteen ironclads and four lighter vessels at the mouth of the Red River on the 7th of March and was joined by a fleet of transport steamers on the 11th. One drawback to this naval operation was the river level. Throughout the winter, the water had been lower than it had been in years, and there was no assurance with a spring melt-off that it would be much higher. Without naval support, taking Shreveport would have required complete repair of the Vicksburg - Shreveport line to bring supplies. Repair would have taken several months, and unless southern Arkansas was purged of Confederate forces, the rail line would be endangered.

After numerous delays, the ground troops reached Alexandria by March 25. Admiral Porter had arrived by that time, and he encountered considerable trouble getting his gunboats over the rocky rapids in the river at Alexandria because of low water. With one force recalled to Vicksburg, another having to guard a supply line from the steamers below the rapids to those above, and a third having to accompany the transports, Banks' army was reduced by 8500 men.

By April 2 and 3, the Army arrived at Natchitoches, roughly half way between Alexandria and Shreveport, and four miles inland from the river town of Grand Ecore. Because of dropping water levels, the larger gunboats could not go further, and the troops aboard the transports had to disembark. The road to Shreveport ran through barren country with little water by way of Pleasant Hill and Mansfield. Although the leading troops had skirmished most of the way, the strategy of Confederate General Kirby Smith was to retreat towards Shreveport, thereby drawing on the Union forces as far as possible before engaging in combat.

The navy had managed with much trouble to reach Springfield, where Banks intended it would establish communications with the land forces at Sabine Crossroads, near Mansfield, and some fifty miles from Natchitoches. On April 7, the first land forces reached Pleasant Hill, where they had driven back a Confederate unit. From that point, a series of blunders occurred. The line of march was strung out twenty or thirty miles, and the forces were not properly marshaled. Then, failure to ascertain Confederate strength and a rash decision to fight occurred. On April 8, a battle took place at Sabine Crossroads, resulting in the Thirteenth Corps and cavalry being routed, with a number of troops taken prisoner and supplies seized. At the end of the day, the 46th counted seven killed, among them Lieutenant Jacob Hudlow, whose commissioning Underhill had noted in January. Thirteen were wounded, including Captain William Pigman, Captain Frank Swigart, one of the compilers of the regimental history, and Captain Henry Snyder, Underhill's mess mate, who was shot in the right leg and carried the ball for the rest of his life. Eighty-six were missing, among them the beloved regimental chaplain, Hamilton Robb, by then in his late sixties, who was captured and with the other prisoners made a forced march of sixteen days with little food or water to Camp Ford, near Tyler, Texas. He was not released until June.

What remained of the regiment retreated to Pleasant Hill, where another battle took place the next day, the Union forces eventually prevailing. But while some officers then called for an advance, others counseled against it, for a variety of sound reasons. Ironically, had Dick Taylor, son of Zachary Taylor, obeyed orders and not engaged Union troops when he did, he might have inflicted far more damage. The Union forces might have been led to Shreveport, far from supply lines, and then set upon by a reinforced Confederate force. As well, the fleet might have been destroyed.

As it was, the fleet had a bad enough time. It had reached a point called Loggy Bayou on April 10, and when the disaster of the army became known, it turned around and made its way back downstream. However, because of worsening water levels, it had to move very slowly and was attacked several times en route. After a difficult passage it eventually reached Alexandria, which the army had reached on April 25 and 26, after it too had been attacked frequently along the way.

Once at Alexandria, the fleet had to traverse the mile of rapids in the river, and a clever means to do this was devised by Lieutenant Colonel Joseph Bailey, a 19th Corps engineer. At the bottom of the rapids, a dam was constructed in the river, and just above it, two wing dams were built. While several thousand men worked on this project from May 2-8, the 46th was in the line of battle, frequently skirmishing, keeping the Confederates at bay. The dam caused the water level in the river to rise over six feet, allowing Admiral Porter to get four gunboats downstream easily. He was a little slow with the others, however, having doubted the merits of the plan, and before he got the rest down, water pressure broke away the works. Additional wing dams had to be built, during which time the 46th was again keeping the Confederates back, but by May 13, the fleet had gotten through, although not without losses because of attacks. The forces then went on to Simmport, on the Atchafalaya River, which they crossed on May 20. General Banks arrived to find that he was to be relieved by General E. R. S. Canby as Commander of the Gulf. Porter made his way back to the Mississippi and resumed river patrol. The 46th arrived at Morganza, Louisiana, above Port Hudson but on the opposite shore of the Mississippi, from which it returned to New Orleans.

The regimental history sums up the disastrous Red River expedition:

> And now the unfortunate Red river campaign was over. An expedition, fitted out with the greatest care and liberality, had come to naught through the neglect of the controlling officers to regard the plainest military rules. Human life, money, and prestige had been sacrificed for nothing.
>
> To the Forty-sixth the campaign had been one of especial hardship and suffering. It marched and fought, almost continuously, from the 6th of March to the 22nd of May. Its members had re-enlisted on the 2d of January, under a general and special promise of a thirty-day furlough home. Most of the men had not seen their families for over two years and a half, but were required to give up the anticipated pleasure and undertake a long, laborious and dangerous campaign. The regiment had marched over 800 miles, much it in the night, and all of it in haste. Comparing the condition of the regiment now with what it was on re-enlistment, the men remembered with sorrow that over a third of their number occupied a rebel prison, the hospital or the grave.[26]

The 46th remained near New Orleans only a short time before it eventually left, after some bureaucratic delays, for Indiana on June 12, 1864 on a long overdue veteran furlough. Although the regiment had an uneventful trip to Cairo, Illinois aboard the *Sultana*, others were not so lucky. On April 1, 1865, a few miles above Memphis, an explosion aboard the *Sultana* blew out one side of the boat. She was carrying nearly two thousand Union soldiers, many former prisoners of war headed for home. Approximately fifteen hundred men were lost. She was the fifth boat to carry that name, and after the disaster, the last.

At Cairo a problem arose when a quartermaster refused to ship six horses belonging to the 46th, but the regiment deliberately made such a nuisance of itself on the river bank that complaints from local people persuaded the quartermaster to ship the unit out! The regiment received warm welcomes in Indiana, both in Indianapolis and in Logansport. For May and June, Underhill is noted on the Field and Staff Muster Roll as absent and is shown on the Detachment Muster Roll as being present in Logansport, Indiana on recruiting service.

On July 20, 1864, the regiment received orders to assemble in Logansport July 26th, which it did, following its furlough, leaving on the 27th for Indianapolis where it remained until August 11th.

The 46th regimental history in the Indiana Adjutant General's report gives its last year or so as follows:

> When about to return to the field, after the expiration of its furlough, the regiment was sent out, first down the Ohio, towards Shawneetown, then through Kentucky to Lexington, to resist the invasion of that State by a rebel force. It marched, under General Burbridge, on an expedition to Saltville, and garrisoned Prestonsburg and Catlettsburg, Kentucky. Returning from this expedition, the Regiment went into garrison at Lexington where it remained until September, 1865.[27]

On the Field and Staff Muster Roll, Underhill is shown as present during September and October 1864, but for November and December, the record merely indicates "not stated." While northern Indiana was

Indianapolis. Aug. 6. 1864

Gen. Noble

Sir:

I can cheerfully reccommend the appointment of Dr. J. W. Underhill as Surgeon of one of the regiments about to be raised.

Dr. Underhill has been with the 46th Regiment in the Medical department ever since its organization. He is now Assistant Surgeon. He is, so far as I can know, well qualified for the position. His experience of the past three years is sufficient to conduct the medical department of a regiment with success.

Dr. Underhill, I am glad to be able to say, possesses none of the vices that so frequently disgrace the service in the person of many of its officers.

Respectfully

T. H. Bringhurst

Col. 46th Regt. Ind. Vet. Vols.

I cordially unite with Col Bringhurst in the above recommendation.

Wm. McLean

Col 43rd Ind Vet Infantry

Underhill had unsuccessfully sought promotion to Surgeon earlier in the war, but in August 1864, in anticipation of the regimental Surgeon mustering out in December 1864, Underhill received the written endorsement of the regiment's Colonel Bringhurst. The promotion would eventually come, but for many months, Underhill would have to wait.

solidly for the war, many in the southern part sympathized with the South and welcomed the Democratic calls for peace. By the summer of 1864, southern Indiana was believed to be a hotbed of Copperheads, Southern sympathizers. The presidential election was coming in November 1864, and Lincoln, running against McClellan, was worried about losing because of poor Union morale during the summer and because of mixed support for his stand on emancipation. Although many states provided for some sort of absentee ballot, Indiana did not. Lincoln viewed the Indiana vote as critical and quietly asked Grant to furlough as many Indiana soldiers as possible so that they could return home to vote. There is virtually no evidence that Underhill did this, and the "not stated" on his presence on the muster roll may be mere administrative oversight. However, Underhill was a Republican, and the possibility exists that he could have gone back.

On December 28, 1864, Underhill's superior, Dr. Israel Washburn, mustered out as regimental Surgeon. After the disappointment of Washburn's having been selected Surgeon ahead of him, Underhill was determined to move up when Washburn left. No one opposed this. In separate letters dated August 6, 1864, both Washburn and Colonel Bringhurst recommended Underhill for the position, since Washburn knew that he would be leaving at the end of December. The bureaucracy must have moved slowly, however, for on January 2, 1865, Bringhurst wrote from regimental headquarters in Lexington, Kentucky to the Adjutant General of Indiana once again recommending Underhill. Then, on January 12, Underhill wrote directly to Governor Morton:

> Sir:
>
> I have the honor to inquire whether any recommendation has been made for a Surgeon to fill the vacancy occasioned Dec'r 28 1864 by the muster=out of Dr. Israel B. Washburn, late Surgeon of the 46 Reg't Ind. Vet. Vol. Inf.? An answer to this would be obligingly received.

> Excuse the irregularity of the request and believe me
> Very respectfully,
> Your ob't Servt.
> J. W. Underhill, Ass't Surg.
> 46 Reg. Ind. Vols.

On January 19, Colonel Bringhurst wrote the Adjutant General once more:

> About twenty days since I sent you a recommendation for the appointment of Asst. Surgeon J. W. Underhill, as Surgeon and of A. B. Herman as 1st Lieut. 46 Regt. Ind. Vet. Vols. I have today received all the other commissions sent for and suppose the letter recommending these above mentioned was lost. I respectfully recommend the appointment of Asst. Surgeon Joshua W. Underhill Surgeon of the 46th Regt. Ind. Vet. Vols. – since Surgeon Israel B. Washburn discharged on expiration of term, December 28, 1864....

When there had been no reply by January 30, Underhill wrote again to Governor Morton:

Gov. O. P. Morton.

Sir.-

I have the honor to make a personal application to your Excellency for the Appointment of Surgeon in our regiment (46' Ind. vol.) to fill the vacancy occasioned Decr 28' 1864 by the muster-out of Dr. I. B. Washburn.

I have served in the regiment since its organization - and as Assistant Surgeon since Decr 30. 1862 - half of which time I have performed the duty of the Surgeon, and am now the only Medical Officer in the command. I am a graduate of a regular medical School, and can, if necessary furnish testimonials of my ability from the Dist. Med. Director, or any Surgeons, civil or military, with whom I am acquainted.

I am informed that our regimental commander (Col. Bringhurst) has twice recommended me for the vacancy - and if other recommendations are required they will be furnished by every commissioned officer of the regiment.

Lexington. Ky. } Very Respectfully
Jany 30 - 1865. } Your Obt Servt.

J. W. Underhill Asst Surgeon
46' Regt Ind vet. vols

After over a month without a regimental Surgeon, on 30 January 1865 a no doubt frustrated Joshua Underhill wrote directly to Indiana's Governor Oliver P. Morton requesting that he might be appointed to that post. Seven days later he received his commission as Surgeon.

Sir:

I have the honor to make a personal application to your excellency for the Appointment of Surgeon in our regiment (46 Ind. Vols.) to fill the vacancy occasioned Dec 28 1864 by the muster=out of Dr. I. B. Washburn.

I have served in the regiment since its organization – and Assistant Surgeon Since Dec 30, 1862 – half of which time I have performed the duty of the Surgeon, and am now the only medical officer in the command. I am a graduate of a regular medical School, and can, if necessary, furnish testimonials of my ability from the Dist. Med. Director, or any Surgeon, civil or military, with whom I am acquainted.

I am informed that our regimental commander (Col. Bringhurst) has twice recommended me for the vacancy – and if other recommendations are required they will be furnished by every commissioned officer of the regiment.

Very Respectfully.
Your Obt. Serv't.

J. W. Underhill Asst Surgeon
46 Regt Ind Vet. Vols.

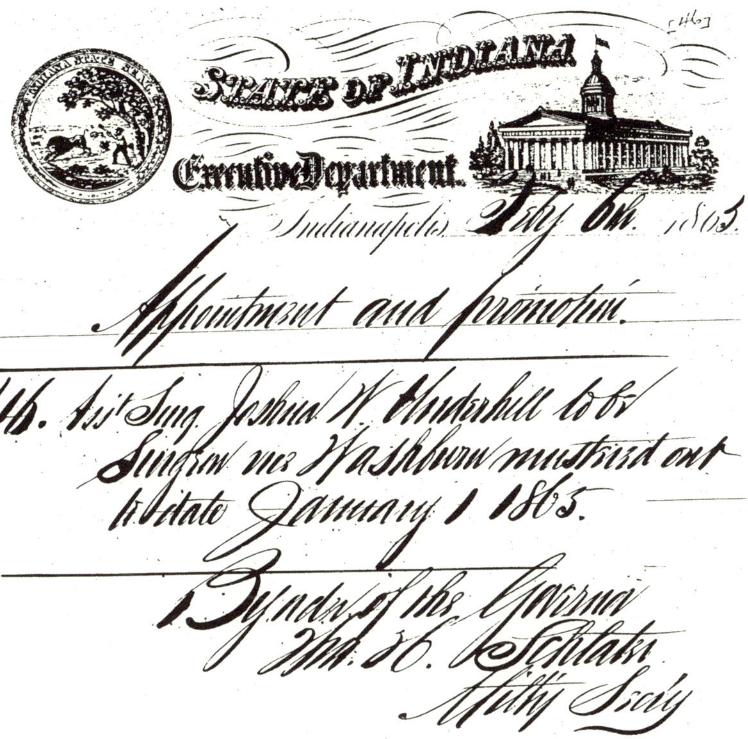

STATE OF INDIANA

Executive Department.

Indianapolis Feby 6th 1865.

Appointment and promotion.

146. Ass't Surg Joshua W. Underhill to be Surgeon vice Washburn mustered out to date January 1 1865.

By order of the Governor
W. H. H. Schlater
Mily Secy

"By order of the Governor," Underhill was promoted from Assistant Surgeon to Surgeon on 6 February 1865. As he had already been performing the role of Surgeon, the promotion was made effective as of 1 January 1865.

Underhill finally got his appointment. The commission from the State of Indiana, Executive Department, is dated February 6, 1865, to date from 1 January 1865, and records note that he officially assumed the duties of Surgeon on February 8.

The regimental Field and Staff Muster Roll shows him as absent from January through May as Post Surgeon, in charge of Prison Numbers 3 and 4, in Lexington, Kentucky. The June roster shows him as transferred per order of Major General Palmer to the Prison Barracks Hospital at Louisville, Kentucky. On July 31, 1865, Underhill filed the following report:

Louisville, Ky.
July 31 - 1865

Sir:

I have the honor to submit the following personal report: Date of Commission January 1st 1865. Serving with my own regiment and also with Detach. of 30 Wis. Vol. Inf. at Market St Barracks since July 6, 1865. To-day (July 31) by verbal order of Post Surgeon in addition to my previous duties report for duty to the Medical Officer in charge of Post Hospital.

Respectfully submitted,
J. W. Underhill
Surgeon 46 Reg. Ind. Vols.

Surgeon Otis Hoyt
30 Regt. Wis. Vol. Inf
Post Surgeon, Louisville Ky.

On September 4, 1865, after submitting this final report to the Medical Director of the Department of Kentucky, Underhill was mustered out out of the service with his regiment:

Louisville, Ky.
Sept. 5 - 1865

Sir:

I have the honor to inform you that I was yesterday mustered out of the Service as Surgeon 46 Reg. Ind. Inf. Vet. Vols., to date Sept 4 - 1865. All medical and hospi-

> tal property in my possession was previously transferred to the Medical Store Keeper, and proper returns made therefor. Should any official matter be addressed to me through the Office of Department Medical Director, it will be received by forwarding to my P.O. address at Logansport, Ind.

After the regiment was mustered out at Louisville, it was transported to Indianapolis, where, on September 11, the men received their final pay. Then, the regiment disbanded:

> And so, the Forty-sixth Regiment Indiana Volunteer Infantry passed into history. Its members having faithfully served their terms of enlistment and reenlisted, were again merged into the citizenship of the Nation. All felt proud of the record of their regiment, for no page of it brought discredit to its members or the State.[28]

Life After the War

When he returned to civilian life, Underhill was nearly twenty-nine and still single. Although he had given a forwarding address in Logansport, Indiana, he did not return to his prewar practice in Burnettsville. Immediately following his discharge, he set off for New York, enrolling in the Bellevue Hospital Medical College, where he attended medical lectures and studied privately with two doctors, Austin Flint and Frank H. Hamilton.

Austin Flint, Sr. (1812-1886) had helped to found and was a professor at the Bellevue Hospital Medical College. A bespectacled, wide-faced man with sideburns and a generous but determined aspect, Flint was descended from a long line of distinguished physicians, receiving his MD degree from Harvard in 1833. He then went to Buffalo where he both practiced and published, and in 1847, helped to found the Buffalo Medical College. In 1861 he moved to New York, where he joined the staff of Bellevue Hospital and also became a professor of the principles and practice of medicine and of clinical medicine at its newly-established medical college. His son, Austin Flint, Jr., also became a distinguished physician and moved with his father.

Vermont-born Frank Hastings Hamilton (1813-1886) graduated from the medical college at the University of Pennsylvania, going in 1833 to Auburn, New York, then in 1844 to Buffalo, where, along with Austin Flint, Sr., he helped to found the Buffalo Medical College. In 1862, following Flint, he moved to New York, where he too served for a period as a professor at the Bellevue Hospital Medical College. Hamilton was a highly distinguished surgeon who not only developed new surgical procedures but also used his considerable engineering talent to modify and invent surgical tools and apparatus.

One of Hamilton's students in Buffalo was Stephen Smith, ten years Hamilton's junior and author of a highly successful book Underhill mentions in his February 18, 1863 diary entry: "... 'Hand Book of Surgery' by Stephen S. Smith Surgeon to Bellvue [sic] Hospital N.Y. An excellent work for Army surgeons." After study in Buffalo, Smith received his MD degree in 1850 at the College of Physicians and Surgeons in New York. With Flint and Hamilton, he too was involved with founding the medical college at Bellevue and was on its faculty while Underhill studied there. After completing his studies in April of 1866, Underhill left Bellevue with an *ad eundem*, or honorary, degree.

In May, he settled in Cincinnati's West End, a crowded section of the city bustling with various medical institutions, breweries, lumber yards, abattoirs, and myriad other businesses. Even along elegant Dayton Street, known as "Millionaires' Row," many houses had raised stoops and iron fences around front yards to keep out pigs sometimes herded along the street on their way to becoming ham and bacon. Local residents were well aware of Cincinnati being "Porkopolis" when the wind came from the wrong direction, and the smell of hops bespoke the nearby breweries.

At 427 John Street, Underhill opened an office with George K. Taylor, who had just completed medical school at Bellevue. Underhill and Taylor remained in practice together until 1869. Why they parted company is not known, but Taylor continued to practice in Cincinnati and in 1893 is shown with an office at 317 Linn Street, a couple of blocks over from John Street.

The houses in the neighborhood were mostly semi-detached or attached brick row houses of two or three stories, many with wooden cornices and wooden back porches, sitting on narrow lots generally about twenty-five feet wide along the street but running a hundred or so feet back allowing for very small back yards. Some houses were single-family, while others contained several apartments. John Street was respectable but not upscale, a solid family neighborhood housing artisans, tradesmen, policemen, office workers, and shopkeepers, along with some lawyers and doctors. Underhill is listed in the city directories as a physician and surgeon, but his specialty was obstetrics and gynecology.

He lived close to the Cincinnati College of Medicine and Surgery, his alma mater. Located first at Longworth and Central Avenues, it later moved to George Street between John and Smith, moving again in 1894, several years after Underhill's death, to Vine Street, above Liberty, where it continued on until 1901, when it was taken into the University of Cincinnati to become part of the present-day Medical College.

Underhill's intellectual bent appears in the diary, not only in his recreational reading, Dickens, Scott, and others, but in the "medical quiz" he and his colleagues engaged in during December 1862 at Helena until troop movements interrupted it, as well as in his studying with such interest Dr. Smith's *Hand Book of Surgery* and what he called "Sargent's Minor Surgery."

Thus it was natural that in the fall of 1866, he joined the College faculty as a demonstrator of anatomy, in charge of the dissecting room. The college was small, its 1872 catalog listing a faculty of only twelve. Faculty turnover was rather high in the early years, but over his years there, Underhill worked with some of Cincinnati's top physicians.

For several years, Thaddeus A. Reamy, eight years older than Underhill, was Professor of Materia Medica (pharmacology) at the college, commuting from Zanesville to Cincinnati to lecture. When Underhill was a student there in 1860-61, he got to know Reamy, and in 1871, Reamy moved to Cincinnati to teach at the Medical College of Ohio. In 1876 he became with Underhill one of the twelve founders of the Cincinnati Obstetrical Society and eventually a most influential member, succeeding Underhill as president in 1880. In a day when babies were primarily delivered by midwives and the presence of a male was considered indelicate, Reamy lobbied vigorously to get medical students into the delivery room as part of their training. Reamy published voluminously and started his own hospital to treat diseases of women. He was a captivating speaker with a quaint sense of humor and a vigorous, encouraging manner that endeared him to students; however, he fearlessly promoted his views and was staunch in a fight, sometimes not endearing himself to some of his colleagues.

Abijah J. Miles, two years older than Underhill, taught pediatrics and gynecology and was on the faculty for some time contemporaneously with Underhill. He, too, was a founder of the Cincinnati Obstetrical Society, along with Swiss-born Jacob Trush, who taught various subjects over the years, including physiology, obstetrics, dermatology, and the principles and practice of medicine and clinical medicine. Trush was highly respected as a lecturer and teacher. For several years before Underhill's arrival on staff and for some years afterward, John A. Thacker taught psychology and diseases of the mind and later principles and practice of medicine and clinical medicine. With rather heavy-lidded eyes and a full white beard and a very long, drooping moustache, Thacker in his photograph appears humorless and melancholy, but he was an eminent medical journalist whose clear thinking, moral courage, and writing skill earned him much respect. In 1877 Joseph Aub joined the faculty as professor of ophthalmology and aural surgery. He was nine years younger than Underhill, the son of Bavarians. He earned his first MD at the Medical College of Ohio and then earned a second in Germany at Erlangen University. A compact man with dark hair, he was a workaholic who burned out early, dying of exhaustion in his early forties, a few months before Underhill.

Underhill held his post as demonstrator of anatomy until 1870, when he was away for two academic years after having been elected Coroner for Hamilton County, with an office downtown at 16 Court House Building, where he is listed in 1871 and 1872. His experience as Hamilton County Coroner gave him considerable expertise in the legal aspects of medicine, and in the fall of 1872, shortly before his term was up, he returned to the Cincinnati College of Medicine and Surgery as a lecturer in medical jurisprudence, the course catalog under this topic carrying the following:

> The services of Dr. J. W. Underhill have been secured to give regular lectures on this interesting and important department of medical education. Dr. Underhill is the present Coroner of Hamilton County, and his qualifications are so well known that it is quite unnecessary to enlarge upon them.

Except that his title as Coroner was given in the past tense in the 1873-1874 catalog, the description was the same, and he held this post for seven years. For the 1879-1880 year, he was Professor of Materia Medica (pharmacology) and Therapeutics and for the next two years Professor of Obstetrics. He continued until 1882, but in the 1882-1883 catalog and subsequent ones, his name no longer appears, although in 1883 for the first time the name of Daniel Webster Clancey does, father of William Power Clancey, who married Underhill's granddaughter Marion Hayward.

In 1876 Underhill joined with eleven others to found the the Cincinnati Obstetrical Society, which remains in existence today as the Cincinnati Obstetrical and Gynecological Society. In 1877 and 1878, Underhill was its first secretary, and in 1879, he became its second president, following Dr. J. J. Quinn, who had been president its first two years. Meetings were held monthly, often at someone's home, at which one member would present a paper to be followed by discussion. Membership was restricted, and a candidate had to have been in practice for five years in Cincinnati before being eligible. On occasion, guests were allowed, and one who attended from time to time in the mid 1880s was a young female physician, Mary Elizabeth Osborn, a distant cousin of Underhill's future son-in-law Philip Hayward. At the time of her untimely death at age forty in 1896, she was considered one of the leading female physicians in the Midwest.

In the Society's Centennial History, written in 1976, Dr. Arthur King wrote: "On November 14, 1878, Joshua W. Underhill gave a paper entitled 'The Female Generative organs in Their Medicolegal Relations' which is not only a classic of medical jurisprudence but of particular value today when almost every medical-legal conference or paper merely repeats what Underhill wrote one hundred years ago." [29]

The discussion following the presentation took over eight pages in the Society's minutes, and the paper itself, printed in *The American Journal of Obstetrics,* took up over seventeen pages.[30]

In addition to his medical practice and teaching, Underhill published a number of highly-respected articles in *The American Journal of Obstetrics,* the *Obstetric Gazette,* the *Cincinnati Medical News,* and the *Lancet and Clinic.*

King writes of him:

> Joshua W. Underhill stood next to Marmaduke Burr Wright in national recognition, and was elected to the limited membership in the American Gynecological Society in 1879. Without question he was the most prolific and far-ranging writer in Cincinnati, and until his later years the most respected.... He had the skill to organize what he had learned and to present it clearly to those who would listen. Finally he had the zeal to contribute his knowledge and experience through numerous publications. His analyses were encyclopedic, thorough, and authoritative.... While not active in politics as such he entered every controversy with a vigor and forthrightness which made him many enemies... and among his colleagues a certain amount of jealousy was apparent...[31]

As well, Underhill also served on the Cincinnati School Board. His preceptor, Dr. McPherson, had served on the school boards in Fairview and Cambridge, and perhaps following McPherson's example, Underhill ran for election and was elected twice from Ward 15, both in April 1876 and again in 1878. In 1880, when twelve members were elected at large, he received the second highest majority of those chosen. He was president of the School Board in 1880 and 1881, and also served as one of the Board of Examiners of teachers.

On June 16, 1874, a big change occurred in Underhill's personal life. The Reverend P. G. Edmonds, minister of the Methodist-Episcopal church in Fairview, Ohio, joined in marriage Underhill and Eliza McPherson, the oldest daughter of his old medical preceptor. Underhill was thirty-seven. Eliza, whose nickname was Lida – although she is "Lyda" on the marriage license – had been born in Fairview and was some twelve years younger. She was from all accounts an earnest, affectionate, highly intelligent, and strong woman. In 1864 she left Fairview to attend Miss Emma Willard's Female Seminary – now the Emma Willard School – of Troy, N.Y. In 1866, the same spring when Underhill finished at Bellevue and settled in Cincinnati, she graduated with honors and was the youngest graduate the school had had up to that time. Before her marriage she taught mathematics for four years at the high school in Princeton, Illinois, where she had gone to live for a time with Judge Henry Kennon, her great uncle. Although the date she returned to Fairview cannot be ascertained exactly, she was there in the fall of 1873. Nothing is known about their courtship, except that Underhill had known the McPhersons well for many years and had known the girls when they were children.

Eliza had two younger sisters: Mary, known as Mollie, born in July 1850, and Jennie, born in March 1857. Jennie had gone to Wesley College in Cincinnati and attended Mt. Holyoke, in Massachusetts. In 1887 she married John Ogier, a Cambridge, Ohio native almost fourteen years her senior, whose family owned a local pharmacy. They remained in Cambridge.

Following Eliza, Mary also attended the Troy Seminary from 1865 to 1869. In 1870 she married William Henry Dunham, originally from St.

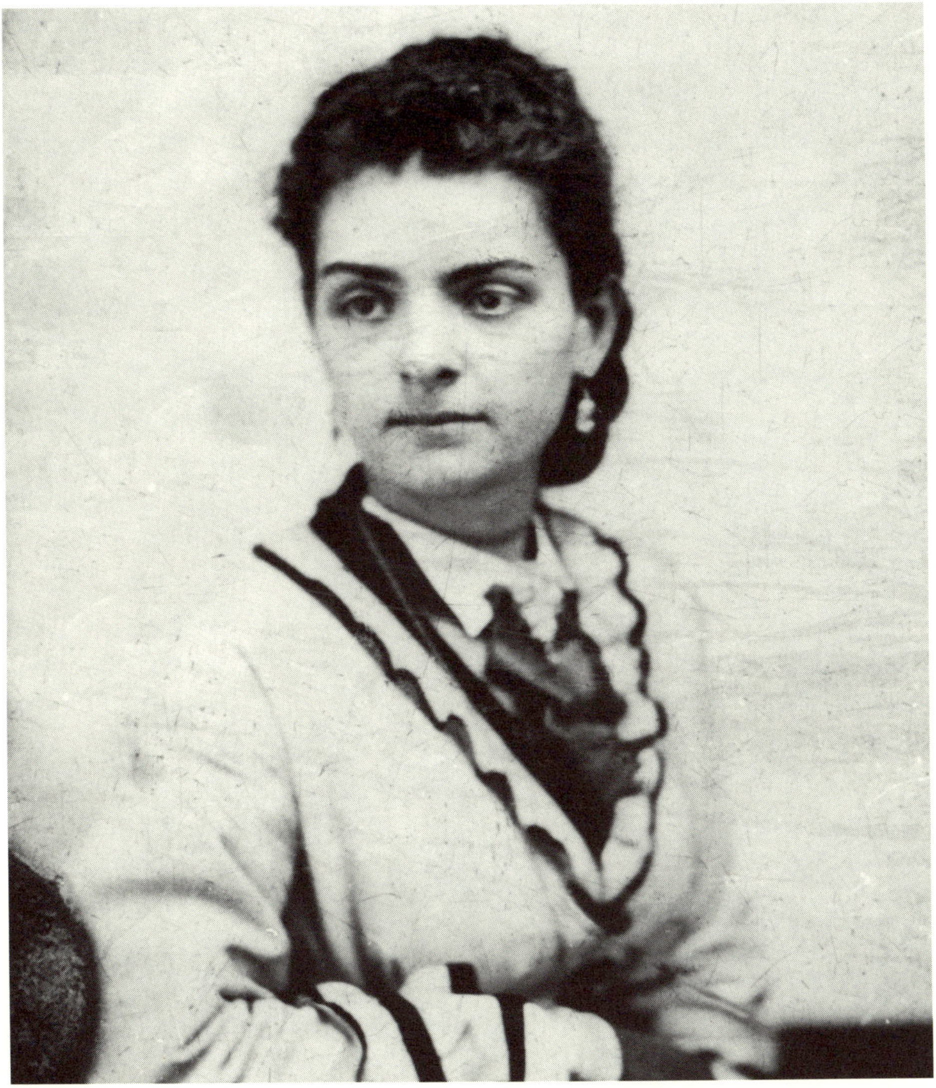

Eliza (McPherson) Underhill (1849-1894) was the oldest daughter of Jeremiah Townsend and Mary (Gilliland) McPerson. After she married Joshua Whittington Underhill on June 16, 1874, in Fairview, Ohio, she lived in Cincinnati, where this photograph was taken about 1883. She died at age forty-five in Cambridge, Ohio in September 1894, leaving three orphaned children.

Clairsville but who had later moved to Fairview. He was five years older. Sometime in the 1860s, Dunham had studied medicine with a preceptor, Dr. A. W. Hewetson of St. Clairsville, and then had gone on to the Starling Medical College but had never taken a degree. For fourteen years he practiced as a licentiate, but in 1879 he went for a year to the Cincinnati College of Medicine and Surgery to complete his MD. Early in 1880, the Dunhams and their two young children were living with the McPhersons in Cambridge, possibly because he had been away in Cincinnati at medical school, but later that year, the Dunhams moved permanently to Cincinnati, to a house at 428 Baymiller Street, at the southeast corner of Findlay Street, which Dr. McPherson appears to have bought for her. In 1882 Dunham went into practice with Underhill, Dunham keeping morning office hours at 418 John Street with Underhill and evening office hours at his own house. Dunham went on to teach therapeutics at the Laura Memorial College and obstetrics at the Cincinnati College of Medicine and Surgery, later helping to organize the Women's Medical College where he was a professor of diseases of children.

The Dunhams had three children: Henry Kennon, born in Fairview in 1872, who later went on to become a successful physician and pulmonary specialist after whom the Dunham Hospital in Cincinnati was named in 1945 following his death; Mary, born in Fairview in 1878, who married Stanley Matthews; and Lida, born in Cincinnati in 1881, who later married Stanley's brother Elijah. The Dunhams remained on Baymiller Street until 1887, when they moved to an elegant stone house, still standing today, with two bow windows and a porte-cochere, at 114 Dayton Street (830 in the modern numbering), for which they paid $15,000. The Dunhams and Underhills lived only a few blocks from each other, and the families knew each other well.

In 1884 Dunham became a member of the Cincinnati Obstetrical Society. On November 8, 1888, Dr. and Mrs. Dunham hosted the Society, and the minutes for the meeting note that "The host of the society for this evening Dr. W. H. Dunham then invited his guests to

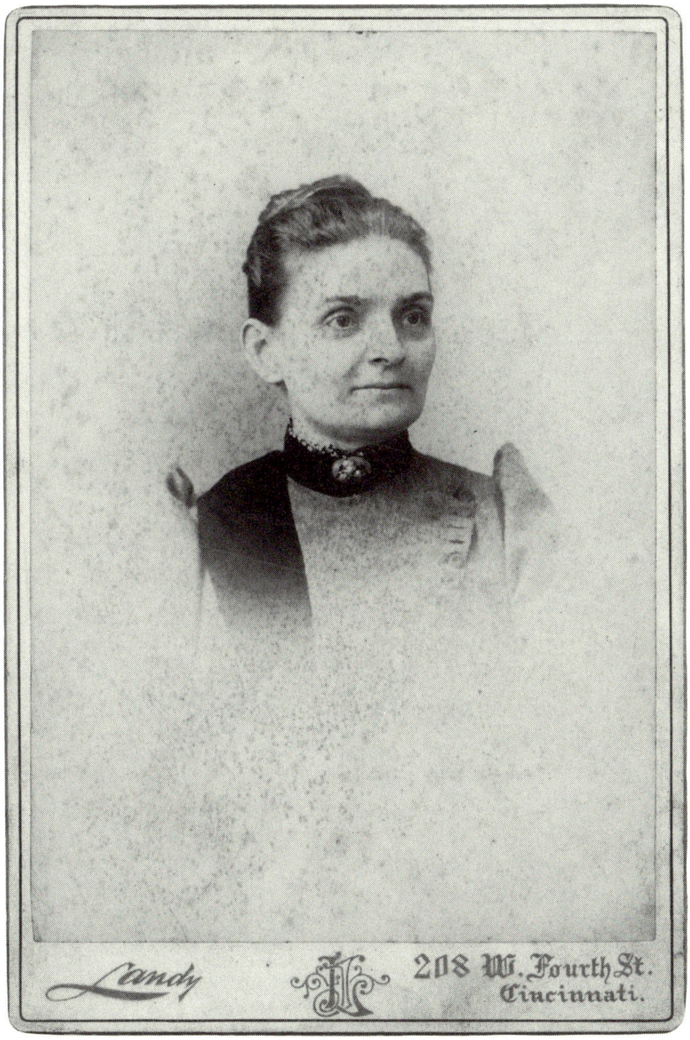

Mary Kennon (McPherson) Dunham (1850-1931) was the middle of the three daughters of Jeremiah Townsend McPherson and Mary (Gilliland) McPherson. She was born a year after Eliza (McPherson) Underhill, the wife of the diarist. Mary married Dr. William Henry Dunham and lived in Cincinnati, Ohio, where this picture was taken during or after 1888. Beginning in 1897, the Underhill children lived with the Dunhams at Cincinnati.

Children of Jeremiah T. and Mary (Gilliland) McPherson

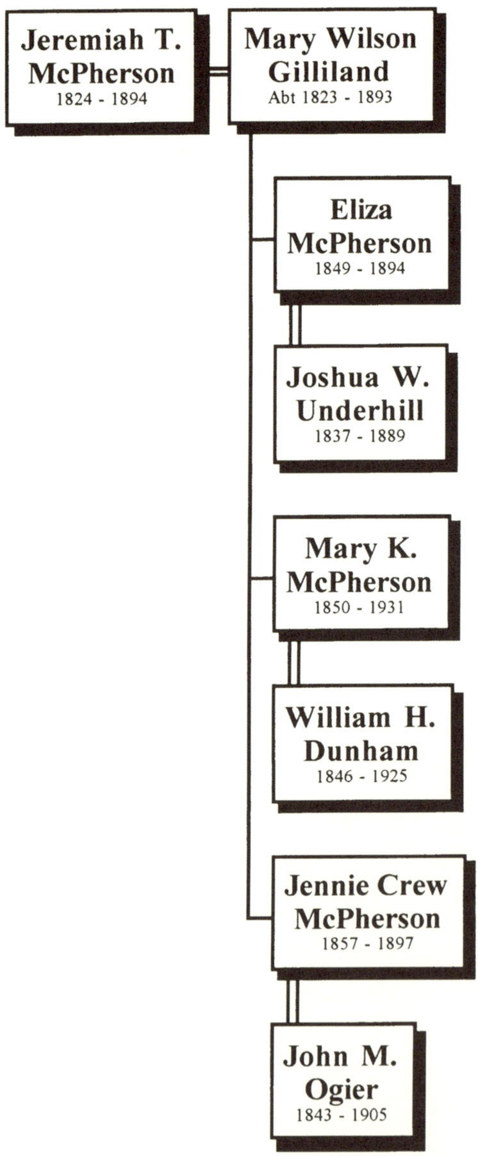

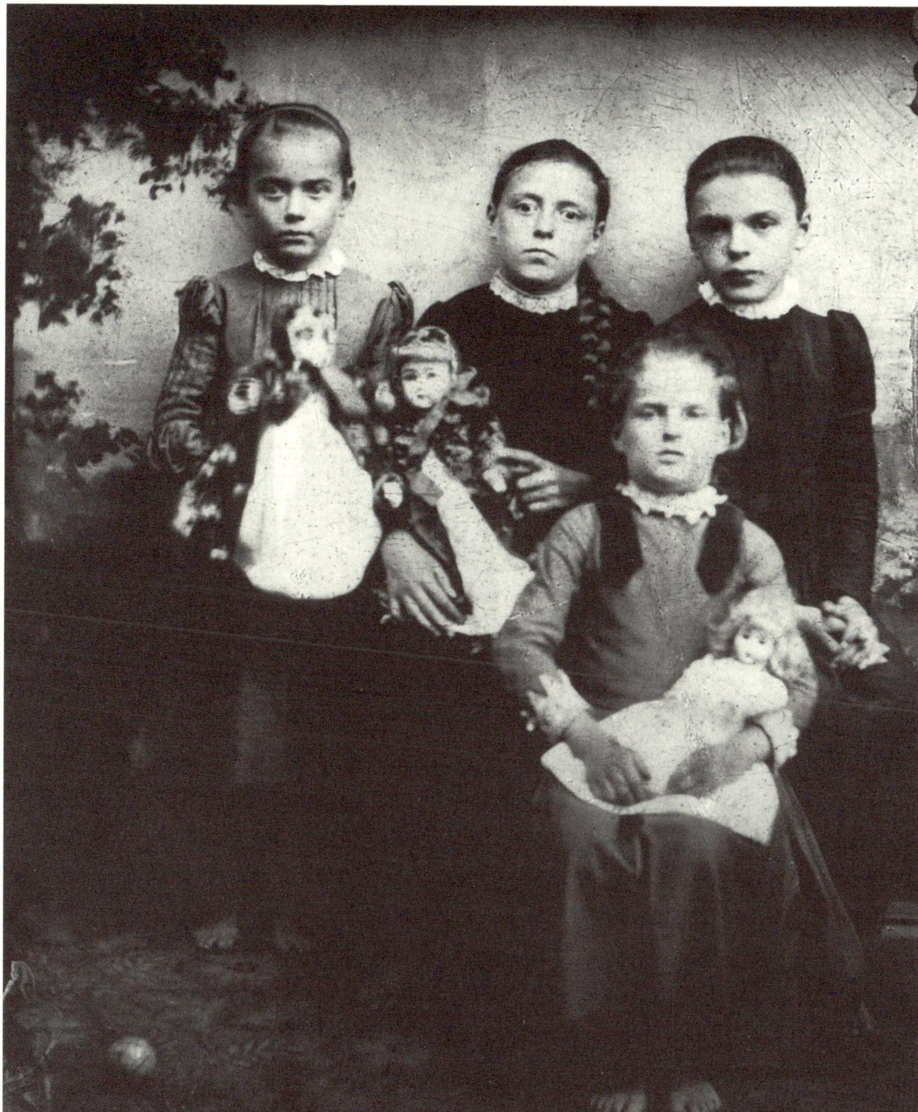

Photographed at Cincinnati in 1886 with dolls in hand were four young Underhill and Dunham cousins: (back row, left to right) Eliza Gilliland Underhill, born 1883; Mary Letitia Dunham, born 1878; Nelle Abbot Underhill, born 1879; and (front row) Lida Jere Dunham, born 1881.

a sumptuous repast spread by his amiable wife in honor of the first meeting of the society in the elegant new residence of the host and hostess. After a convivial hour spent in this manner, adjourned."

In 1870 Underhill had moved to 432 John Street, but by mid-November 1873, Underhill was living at 434 John Street, a single family house where he brought his bride and where their first three children were born. Mary Eleanor was the oldest, born August 4, 1875, and named for both grandmothers. Their only son, Whittington Townsend Underhill, was born December 29, 1876. Nelle Abbot Underhill arrived July 28, 1879. Also living with them by the middle of 1880 was a nineteen year old servant girl named Lulu McTon.

On October 6, 1880, Frederick C. Tucker granted Underhill a five year lease on a detached single-family house at 26 Clinton Street where Tucker had been living with his two brothers. The rent was $300 per year, payable quarterly, and Underhill was to pay as well all taxes and assessments and to maintain the property at his expense. He also had the option to buy the house for $7000. It was just around the corner from the Underhills' old house, and on one side it looked out across an alley to the small back yards behind houses along John Street and on the other at a Presbyterian church. Here Jean Underhill was born on February 25, 1882 and Eliza Gilliland Underhill, the youngest, on June 18, 1883.

Sadly, though, two of the girls did not live long. At 3:30 AM on April 15, 1881, Mary Eleanor, after being ill for three weeks with typho-malarial fever and in the end, with cerebral meningitis, died four months before her sixth birthday. Dr. William Carson, Underhill's colleague on the staff of the Cincinnati Hospital, a dour man but highly respected as an excellent diagnostician, could not save her, and his signature appears on the death certificate. Her funeral was held at the house the next afternoon and she was buried privately at Spring Grove in a lot owned by Mary McMurphy, a widowed sixty year old, English-born neighbor who lived close by on Everett Street with her son Theodore, a special agent for the Aetna Insurance Company. Mary

Children of Joshua W. and Eliza (McPherson) Underhill

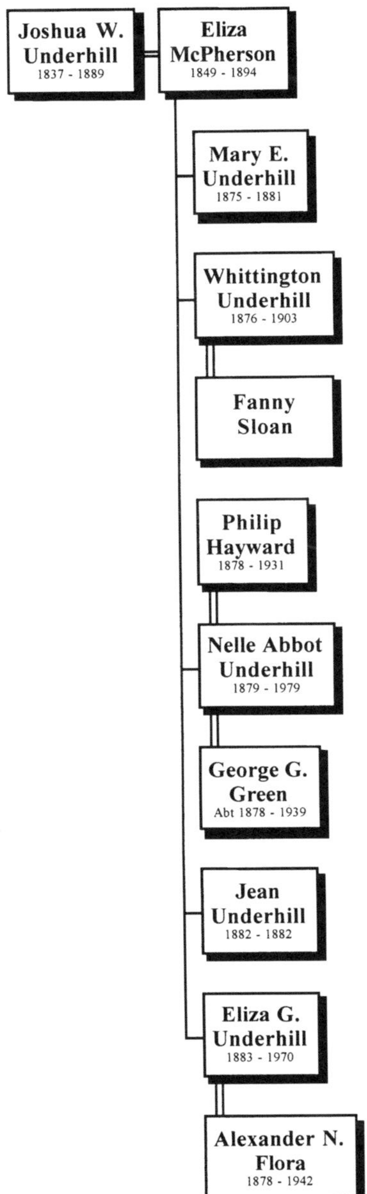

Eleanor's death was a crushing blow from which Underhill never recovered.

The next year, on November 1, 1882, Carson had to sign another death certificate. Jean Underhill, at the age of nine months, died after a week's illness, the cause of death shown as acute pneumonia and ultimately, congestion of the brain (probably encephalitis). Her funeral was held at the house at two o'clock the following day, after which she joined her sister at Spring Grove.

Devastating as these deaths were, they were common. At that time in Cincinnati, one child in three did not live beyond a first birthday. Doctors and health officials of the period were plagued with problems largely overcome in the modern day. Tuberculosis, lung infections, typhoid fever, encephalitis, meningitis, and diphtheria were common diseases. Dr. J. J. Quinn, Underhill's predecessor as President of the Cincinnati Obstetrical Society, served from 1873 to 1876 as Health Officer to the city. An early crisis he faced was controlling an outbreak of cholera in 1873. He lobbied hard for proper sewerage, and one successor pushed for adequate filtration of the city water supply, services taken for granted today.

But life had to continue, and it did. Both Joshua and Eliza Underhill were strong. They picked themselves up, rejoiced in the good health of their three surviving children, and carried on. But life as they had known it was to last only several years more, until an especially insidious demon invaded their lives. Joshua Underhill became addicted to cocaine.

The Final Period

How Joshua Underhill became addicted to cocaine has not been definitively established. The chronology of the last several years of Underhill's life comes largely from the January 29 and 30, 1889 issues of *The Cincinnati Enquirer*, (published over the two days following his death) which presented two conflicting explanations for his addiction. The January 29 edition carried the following:

> [Underhill] told a curious tale about his becoming addicted to the habit to a number of persons, and what truth, if any, there is in it is for the public to judge. He was at one time a Director of the Cincinnati Hospital, and about the time the anaesthetic quality of cocaine was discovered (in 1884) some leading physicians, he said, wished to try the experiment on him. He was hale and healthy, had no constitutional disease, no hereditary taint of indiscretions of former generations, was possessed of great firmness of character and will-power, so he was induced to try cocaine.[32]

The January 30 edition quoted Dr. Abijah J. Miles, Underhill's colleague at the Cincinnati College of Medicine and Surgery, who offered another explanation:

> The case was a most remarkable one. I knew the doctor

> well, and the strange part of it is that a man who was so strong a temperance man should succumb to the habit. He never touched liquor, not even native wine. I recollect that when we had the professors' lunch that Dr. Aub gave we had some Rhine wine and native wines, and the doctor would not touch a drop. Why, he wouldn't even smoke, but held a cigar in his mouth and chewed at the end. I think he had pulmonary trouble, in fact, know he had hemorrhages, and began the use of morphine to ease his pain. He even took a trip to the Bermudas and Florida for his health, and I presume when the morphine habit grew on him he tried cocaine as an antidote. His case is a sad one. He was a bright man and had a glorious future before him.[33]

Whatever the truth about when and how he became addicted, the period leading up to his death was frightening for him and heartbreaking for his family. In an era before the Federal Drug Administration and drug cartels, Underhill was able to obtain small doses of cocaine easily and inexpensively, and as a doctor, he had hypodermic syringes.

Two years before his death, his behavior become noticeably erratic. A clue emerges in the Cincinnati City Directory of 1886, where Dunham, Underhill's partner with whom he had been in practice since 1882 and a member of the family, appears separately. By this time Underhill was addicted and no longer able to practice, and clearly Dunham realized that he could no longer work with Underhill and thus withdrew to practice independently at his home on Baymiller Street.

According to the newspaper, sometime late in 1885 or in 1886, when Underhill's behavior had become increasingly unpredictable, his family sought some way to restrain him and get him off the cocaine. They called in his old friends and colleagues, Thaddeus Reamy and William Carson, who saw to it that an attendant took charge of him, whereupon Underhill reportedly rebelled and fled across the river to Newport,

Kentucky, where he sent for his lawyers and told them that there the Ohio courts could not do anything to him, that he would not return, and that a plot was afoot to put him in an asylum.

The substance abuser does not welcome being confronted about his problem. Under normal circumstances, Underhill was warm and gentlemanly, but he had a temper and was not one to run from a fight, and he proved hopelessly stubborn in the face of all that his family and friends were trying to do to help him. Two other colleagues, John Thacker and Jacob Trush, went to see him, but to no avail. He did return to Cincinnati, but about two years before he died, Eliza Underhill could live with him no longer and left with the children to live with her parents in Cambridge, Ohio.

The newspaper reported that he suffered terrifying hallucinations, imagining monsters and demons after him. The last entry in his diary, made on January 15, 1889, the only one appearing after his November 15, 1873 entry noting getting the diary back, is also its most cryptic: "Bright morning. My Friend were quiet last night comparatively." What appears to be the word *friend* is hard to read. Did Underhill indeed intend *friend*, or did he intend *fiend?* He had two tenants at 418 John Street: Leon Marks, a carpet renovator and manufacturer of melophine, probably akin to benzine for use in carpet cleaning; and Miles Beatty, a plasterer, who, according to the newspaper, watched after Underhill in his last illness. Were they customarily noisy tenants who might have disturbed him at night and might he have meant *friend* in reference to them? Or, if referring to the demons that plagued him, did he intend *friend* ironically? Or was he not being ironic and intended *fiend?* We shall never know. Two weeks later, he was dead.

Underhill died at his home in Cincinnati, by then 418 John Street, at noon on Monday, January 28, 1889. Dr. William H. Wenning's death certificate, as well as the cemetery record at Spring Grove, shows tetanus and resultant lockjaw as the immediate cause of death, the "remote or predisposing" cause as "cocaine habit and slight injury of ankle." The story given out was that a few days before he died, Underhill had dropped a rusted silver-plated fork with enough force that one prong punctured his right ankle. No blood came from the wound, but later the limb began to swell and blood poisoning set in. He was just fifty-two.

Dr. William H. Dunham took charge, calling in the undertaking firm of J. F. Wiltsee. Mrs. Underhill came immediately to Cincinnati from her home in Cambridge, and on Wednesday, January 30, an eleven o'clock funeral service was held at the chapel at Spring Grove Cemetery. Underhill was first buried with Mary and Jean in the lot owned by Mary McMurphy, but on April 7, 1893, he and Mary and Jean were moved to their final resting places in Lot 48, Section 88, a large plot at Spring Grove that Dr. Dunham and Mrs. Underhill had subsequently bought.

Underhill's daughter Nelle once commented rather matter-of-factly that her father had died of drug addiction. In a style considerably less matter-of-fact, the tragic story of his prolonged downfall unfolded in *The Cincinnati Enquirer* for two days following his death. On Tuesday, January 29, the day after he died, bold, lurid headlines were layered down the left column of the front page above his picture:

> COCAINE'S VICTIM. Sad Death of Dr. Underhill. He Succumbs to the Power of the Fatal Drug. Lockjaw Results From His Enfeebled Condition. Dying Deserted By His Wife and Children. The Unfortunate Man Hounded by Hallucinations. How He Fell Into the Clutches of His Insidious Enemy. Pitiful Close of a Bright, Honorable, and Useful Career. His Record as a Soldier, Physician and City Official – Conspicuous Traits of Character.[34]

On Wednesday, January 30, the story had moved to page five but remained a long feature story:

> DR. UNDERHILL. More Facts In Relation to His

> Sad Death. He Refused to Submit to the Orders of His Physicians. And Fled to Kentucky to Secrete Himself From Them. His Uncontrollable Desire for the Dread Drug Cocaine. Was Brought About Through the Use of Morphine for Medicine. Interesting Interviews With Prominent Physicians of This City Regarding the Drug and Its Artificial Manufacture.[35]

Cincinnati then had a population of just under 300,000. The Underhills and Dunhams were cultured and refined, and in a day when convention was strictly observed, one can only imagine their mortification at finding the family scandal blazoned over the front page of the newspaper in yellow journalism.

A man of such self discipline and moral uprightness as Underhill must have been vastly angry and sad at his plight. Carson, along with Thacker and Trush, had long since seen that nothing could be done. Reamy had not seen him for a year. In the spring of 1888, Dr. Wenning had been summoned and without success advised Underhill to go to a sanitarium. In his last illness, Wenning, along with Dr. Burhans, simply gave Underhill sedatives to relax muscle spasms, and after he died, Wenning signed the death certificate. One might assume that in the absence of Mrs. Underhill, Dunham had kept a watchful eye on her husband throughout his travails.

Besides enduring the embarrassment of Underhill's scandalous end, the family suffered as well from financial ruin that emerged after it. On January 31, 1889, the day after Underhill's funeral, Dr. Dunham and Mrs. Underhill appeared before Hamilton County Probate Judge Herman Goebel, seeking Dunham's appointment as administrator of the estate. Mrs. Underhill wrote a statement waiving her right, requesting that Dunham be appointed instead. Dunham signed a statement that to his knowledge, Underhill had left no will but had an estate estimated at $250 in personal property and $8000 in real estate. Dunham nominated George C. Witt, L.W. Fechheimer, and Charles F. Klayer appraisers.

On February 9, in what must have come as a surprise, Underhill's lawyer and an old family friend, J. William Johnson, filed for probate a paper purporting to be Underhill's last will and testament with a codicil. Later in February or very early in March, a hearing was held, and on March 4 the testimony of witnesses was filed. Although neither the purported will nor the transcript of the testimony remain on file with the court, the testimony must have been lengthy, for the stenographer's bill was fifty-three dollars. On March 14 the court handed down a ruling, refusing the will for probate on the ground that Underhill was not of sound mind when he signed it. Johnson stated that he would appeal the ruling, and did so on March 15. What happened to the appeal does not appear in Underhill's estate file with the court, but Johnson must have lost, since Dunham was ultimately appointed administrator.

The three appraisers were sworn in on March 20. All had been neighbors of Underhill. George Witt, almost forty, had been a gauger who lived a block away on Everett Street but was by then a partner in the Witt Cornice Company on Broadway. Bavarian-born Leopold Fechheimer, in his early fifties, was a solicitor for The Mutual Life Insurance Company of New York who lived at 423 John Street. Charles F. Klayer, close to forty, and the American-born son of German immigrants, ran the drugstore at 422 John Street, on the corner of John and Clinton Streets. The final inventory was attested to by Dr. Dunham on May 1 before Judge Goebel. It was discouraging.

Dr. McPherson owed Underhill $500. There was a set of post-mortem and other instruments, damaged, valued at $10. An open-face watch was valued at $15. A list of back accounts showed some fifty patients owing money. Of a total of $1104.25 due, all but $83.50 was considered bad or uncollectable. The appraisers did not even bother appraising the furnishings, which they found in such badly damaged condition that they simply released them to Mrs. Underhill. They also provided her $1800 in cash to support her and the three surviving children for a year, "there being no other suitable property." No mention was made of insurance policies or bank accounts.

As King pointed out, "[Underhill's] private practice was never large or lucrative."[36] Money seems to have been a chronic problem. While much of the time he lived in rented houses, on October 3, 1876, he bought the house at 418 John Street, shown in records as a "tenement," from M. Adelia and Henry V. Wilson for $3720. It had three apartments and he seems to have used it solely as an income property until he moved out of 434 John Street late in 1880. At that time he may have not have had room or wanted his practice at 26 Clinton Street and took over one of the apartments at 418 John Street for his office. By 1885 he was living there as well, the lease on the Clinton Street house having expired. Over the course of seven years he and his wife took out five mortgages on the property.

On May 23, 1878, they got a mortgage from Aaron Klein for $2500, paid back in February 1883. The second, for $2000, granted by Elizabeth Curtis, was taken out in July 1879 and paid back by June 1882. The third, for $2500, granted by the Texas Building Association in June 1882, was paid back three years later, in August 1885. The next, taken out in January 1883 for $2000, granted by Maggie Conrad and payable in two years, was entered as paid on August 6, 1885. On that same date, the Underhills took out the fateful last mortgage for $7000, granted by Charles Meis. It appears as if the Underhills kept getting new mortgages in order to satisfy old ones.

Because Underhill had not worked in several years, and because the income from his two rental units was insufficient to pay the debt, the $7000 mortgage taken out on 418 John Street in 1885 could not be paid. On October 5, 1888, the mortgagee had filed in court for foreclosure and sale of the property. In the March term of the court, Underhill having died in January, his wife and children as heirs and Dunham as his administrator were named defendants in the case. On May 17, a court order was issued to sell the property at auction, and on June 22, at a sale on the premises, someone named Charles Weber was the highest bidder at $7700. In Cambridge on July 18, 1889, in what must have been a humiliating moment, Mrs. Underhill, in the presence of her then aging father and William S. Dougherty, a justice of the peace, deeded the house to Weber for one dollar. Ten weeks later, Weber sold the house to John Theodore Shale for $8500.

Underhill was highly respected, personally, professionally, and for his civic contributions, but in addition to losing two adored children, he seems not to have fully recovered from the war, because for the rest of his life, he appears to have suffered from chronic medical problems which he felt were war-related. On May 4, 1887, nineteen months before he died, Underhill filed a formal application – written by someone else but which he signed – for an invalid pension. He contended that near Fort Pillow in March 1862 he suffered

> ...from exposure and fatigue in line of duty, on a Mississippi River steamer he contracted Malarial Fever and Chronic Diarrhoea, totally disabling him at the time and resulting in Piles, Fistula, and a disease of the Lungs, which finally manifested itself in a hemorrhage of the lungs on or about May 21, 1863 while in the rear of Vicksburg, Miss. and he subsequently have [sic] other hemorrhages during the remainder of his term of service... that July 5, 1863, while under the command of Gen Sherman on the march from Vicksburg to Jackson Miss. he was attacked by a partial sunstroke due to fatigue and extreme heat disabling him at the time and laying the foundation for a migrain [sic] that has returned at intervals of one to three weeks ever since.

He also stated he was treated by Surgeon Coleman on a hospital boat on the Mississippi River for four months in 1862. He went on to say that he was now "totally disabled from obtaining his subsistence by manual labor by reason of his injuries...," inability to perform manual labor being the criterion for establishing disability.

Several of his diary entries record illnesses. On March 31, 1863 he says, "Was quite sick yesterday suffering from nervous headache." On April 21, on the march from Milliken's Bend, Underhill notes, "Been rather unwell since we came here – suffering from nervous debility." On June 17, while in the rear of Vicksburg, he writes, "Have been quite unwell the last few days but managed to perform my duties. Am a little better this morning." Underhill claimed that his first lung hemorrhage occurred about May 21, although nothing to this effect appears in the diary. On July 5 and 6, 1863, he was miserable. On the 5th, he "Was very sick to-day compelled to stop a few hours on the march and rest in the shade." On the 6th, he wrote, "Been lying under the shade of the oak trees resting all day." The weather had been crushingly hot. Clearly this was his partial sunstroke on the march from Vicksburg to Jackson, when he simply could not march with the regiment. Although he claims that his sunstroke on the march to Jackson had precipitated his later migraines, his March 31 entry noting his nervous headache and his April 21 entry noting "nervous debility," which he does not define but which might be construed as a headache, suggest that he may have experienced and been susceptible to bad headaches before suffering the sunstroke.

On September 28, 1887, the Adjutant General's office at the War Department sent a report to the Commissioner of Pensions that a review of Underhill's records had furnished "no evidence of disability while an enlisted man." A further report dated December 30, 1887 noted that "regimental records furnish no evidence of disability in his case while a commissioned officer." It appears that Underhill did not pursue his application any further.

After his death, however, in March 1890, Mrs. Underhill revived the claim. The claim was approved, dating from May 4, 1887 and ending with his death, for malarial poisoning, chronic diarrhoea and resulting disease of rectum, disease of lungs, and sunstroke. He was granted sixteen dollars per month which was increased to twenty-four dollars when the additional disabilities of vertigo and headache were added. The lump sum was payable to her. Starting July 10, 1890, Mrs. Underhill was entitled as well to a pension under the Act of June 27, 1890 of eight dollars per month and two dollars more for each minor child.

But she was in financial straits, and under what appears a different set of provisions she applied in February 1890 for an additional widow's pension. The bureaucracy moved slowly, and an internal Pension Bureau form notes that on May 24, 1890, her congressman, John A. Caldwell, had made enquiries about her application and was to be kept informed. Her cousin, George E. Gilliland, a newspaperman originally from Ohio living in Washington and no doubt well acquainted with the Ohio congressional delegation, had also made enquiries.

While she had been able to show that Underhill's maladies were service-related and thus collect his invalid pension, she then had to convince the authorities that his death was service-related. From January through December 1890, she assembled several affidavits – now in the National Archives – attesting to her husband's illness and disability. The first came from Israel Washburn, whom Underhill had relieved as regimental surgeon, who noted in a physician's affidavit that "Underhill had a severe attack of malarial fever contracted about May 1st 1862 at or near Osceola, Arkansas... [and] was sick about one month. The case was complicated with liver disease as he showed the worst case of Jaundice ever seen by deponent...Underhill had another attack of malarial fever during the month of August 1863 while at Natchez, Miss."

Another was from one of Underhill's regimental mess mates, Captain Henry Snyder, then age fifty-two and living in Monticello, Indiana, a sometime speller who was blunt:

> I was Capt of Co E 46 Regt Ind vol Inft Vet and was well acquainted with Dr. J W Underhill while in the service and in line of duty he contracted cronic diarhea at Helena Ark 1862 and on the march from Jackson Miss to Vicksburg he was attacked by a partial sun stroke due to fatigue and exposure and extreme heat totally disabling him for some time. I have seen him have hemorrhages of the lungs and he was constantly coufing and

> spitting this comenst July 1863 while in rear of Vicksburg Miss. I know the above by being a mess mate of his all the time we was in the service from Oct 13 1861 to May 1864 when I was at Alexandria La I left the Regt by being wounded. I saw Dr. Underhill in 1870 he told me he was still suffering with his lungs.

The pension authorities still felt they needed further evidence and asked several of the affiants for additional information. In an additional statement requested by the government dated June 16, 1891, Snyder recalled that "Joshua W Underhill was Sun Stroke on the march from Jackson to Vicksburg Miss July 1863. My Ricolection is that he had headache and he could not gow in the sun with out an umbrerel. Alwas had Sick headache could not eat expectorated a grate deal got Sore in his lings and was very much unde the weather."

Initial affidavits and affidavits of additional evidence were submitted as well by Thaddeus Reamy, William H. Wenning, and Charles A. Burhans. Reamy found him suffering from nervous headaches, chronic dysentery, and hemorrhoids, and was specific about the postwar problems while acquainted with Underhill after 1871:

> He repeatedly informed me that his severe attacks of headache which recurred every few weeks were due to sunstroke incurred in the service. I have frequently called to see him at his house and found him in bed with these attacks.
>
> The same is true as to his attacks of diarrhoea of which he suffered severely and frequently during the whole time from 1871 until January 1888 [when Reamy no longer saw him]. He also...suffered during this period two different winters...of severe cough with emaciation [sic] and copious expectoration of mucus of purulent character, sometimes bloody.

Dr. W. H. Wenning, another member of the Cincinnati Obstetrical Society, wrote that

> [in the five years before his death, Underhill] frequently informed me that he had repeated attacks of malaria and nervous headache which originated during his service in the army...[In the fall of 1887] I found him suffering from extreme nervous prostration and emaciation. He referred me to the slight attacks of cough which, he feared, were due to lung trouble. On examination I found partial consolidation of the left lung. He also had occasional attacks of diarrhoea. His previous symptoms were undoubtedly due, in a great measure, to the cocaine habit which he had contracted by this time; but it is my firm belief that he had acquired this habit by resorting to the drug in the first instance to overcome temporarily his attacks of debility and bad feeling. I therefore believe that he was totally disabled for manual labor some years previously....

Dr. Charles A. Burhans along with Wenning attended Underhill in his last illness. He was sixteen years younger than Underhill, and for several years while he was attending the Medical College of Ohio, he and his widowed mother Sarah were tenants of Underhill at 418 John Street, although Burhans had first met him at the age of thirteen in 1866. Underhill was a mentor to Burhans, who was thirty by the time he finished at medical school. Burhans

> ...once saw him have a chill in 1866 or 1867, said by attending physician to be Congestive chill; have seen him repeatedly with ordinary chills which were followed by intense sick headaches. Have repeatedly seen him suffering from malaria. Also known that he had piles

> and a fistula which gave him great annoyance, these two troubles were caused by ... diarrhoea... Dr. Underhill had lung trouble and...his expectoration was at times streaked with blood. I remember that at one time he was under the care of Dr. William Carson for pneumonia. His migraine frequently caused him to fail to attend to his business or keep his appointments.

All went on to say that Underhill for some time had been disabled for manual labor and judged his illnesses to be war-related.

Among the documents with her application, Mrs. Underhill filed an Affidavit that the Claimant has not Re-married, and that She is without other means of Support than her Daily Labor. In addition to the printed statement, there is an additional, handwritten statement: that "she is dependent upon others not legally bound to support her, that she has no property of any kind or description whatsoever and further ... the children of said claimant for which pension is claimed are all living, to wit Whittington T., Nellie, and Eliza G. Underhill." The affidavit was signed by her father and her brother-in-law John Ogier.

In the end, her application was rejected December 30, 1891 on the grounds "That Soldiers death from tetanus was not due to his military service as set forth in an official letter from the Commissioner of Pensions and dated Sept. 26, 1892."

Early in October 1892 she filed an appeal with the Secretary of the Interior for a reconsideration of her claim

> ...because she believes that she has shown by competent testimony that the death of her late husband was indirectly due to disability contracted during his military service. She has shown by reputable testimony that her said late husband...because so painfully afflicted from disease contracted in the United States military service that he was compelled to resort to the use of alleviating

> medicines and it appears that the premediate cause of his death was due to the use of drugs which he had resorted to with the hope of relieving him from suffering caused by disease contracted in his military service and in the line of his duty. Claimant has no doubt but that the cause of her late husband's death was remotely due to his military service and if there is a doubt about such being true she asks for the benefit of such doubt.

On July 21, 1893, the Commissioner of Pensions referred the matter to the Secretary of the Interior:

> Feby. 26, 1890, appellant filed an application for pension under the general law, as the widow of Joshua W. Underhill, alleging that the said Joshua W. Underhill died Jany. 28, 1889, of a disability contracted while in the military service.
>
> The claim was rejected Dec. 30, 1891, on the ground that the death cause was not due to disabilities contracted in the service.
>
> The soldier was pensioned to the date of his death for "malarial poisoning, chronic diarrhoea and resulting disease of rectum, disease of lungs, and sunstroke."
>
> The evidence seems to show that he died of convulsions (tetanus) due to the cocaine habit, having taken the drug on this occasion for a slight injury of ankle.
>
> The contention in the appeal is that the soldier was compelled to resort to the use of drugs for the purpose of alleviating the pain caused by his disabilities contracted in the service, and that therefore the soldier's death, from the use of said drugs, was remotely due to his military service.
>
> Appellant was pensioned under the Act of June 27,

> 1890, from July 10, 1890.
>
> The appeal and papers in the case are respectfully submitted for your consideration.

On October 26, 1893, John M. Reynolds, Assistant Secretary of the Interior, replied to the Commissioner of Pensions in a very stiff letter. After a brief review of the case, he then went on:

> Since July 10, 1890, Mrs. Underhill has been drawing a pension under the new law.
>
> As shown by the evidence appellant's husband died at Cincinnati, O., January 28, 1889, the remote or predisposing cause of death being the cocaine habit, and the immediate cause acute tetanus brought on by a slight injury of the right ankle. In an affidavit subscribed by the attending physician, the opinion is expressed that the patient contracted the unfortunate habit in the first instance by resorting to the drug "to overcome his attacks of debility and bad feeling." There is evidence showing that the sunstroke for which Dr. Underhill was in part pensioned subjected him to frequent and severe sick headaches, and the physician referred to above states that said sunstroke would in great measure account for the patient's extreme nervousness.
>
> The contention of the appeal is that the husband was compelled to use drugs to alleviate pain, and that as said pain was caused by disease contracted in the army death from such use is to be considered as remotely due to the military service.
>
> Himself a physician, familiar with the properties of drugs, and aware of the danger to be apprehended from their improper use, appellant's husband cannot be held blameless under the state of facts shown here. It does

> not appear that at any time while he was acquiring the fatal habit Dr. Underhill was enfeebled in mind so as to be incapable of exercising an intelligent professional judgment as to the proper use of a dangerous drug. The fact that he was a physician but added to his responsibility and in the eye of the law rendered his act the more inexcusable. Knowing that cocaine if constantly taken, was ruinous to health, and destructive of life he persisted in its use, regardless of the ultimate consequences and intent only on immediate relief.
>
> If...death be accepted as an incident of the cocaine habit, and that habit as an incident or result of the treatment, we encounter this obstacle, that appellant's husband acquired the fatal habit under treatment which, as carried out, was obviously improper, and for which, it being his own, he alone was responsible.
>
> Rejection affirmed.

Mrs. Underhill continued to receive the original pension and money for each child, but there was no raise in her benefits.

The affidavits that Eliza Underhill filed have a similar, orchestrated quality to them. Destitute, and undoubtedly humiliated by the scandal surrounding her husband's death as well as by having burdened her aged parents with herself and her three children, her desperate attempt to portray her husband's medical condition in the bleakest terms possible in order to get a pension is wholly understandable. The several doctors had been not only colleagues but friends of Underhill, and Henry Snyder was an old Army buddy. They were no doubt glad to do whatever possible to help. Of all the affidavits, Israel Washburn's is the most cautious, but this is to be expected, given what may have been a frosty relationship after their jockeying for promotion to regimental surgeon and that Washburn probably had not seen Underhill since the war and thus could not comment on his later condition. Given the reputations of those who wrote the affidavits, it seems altogether unlikely that fraud was involved, but hyperbole may have been, since the affidavits describe a man almost totally disabled. This may have been the case after Underhill began using cocaine, but before that, he taught ably at the medical school, wrote scholarly articles, was active in professional organizations, carried on a medical practice, was married and produced five children, got elected Hamilton County Coroner, and served for some years on the Cincinnati School Board. Given his many accomplishments and the possibility that the newspaper account of his claim to having been hale and healthy at the time he began using cocaine has any truth, we are faced with two quite different views of his condition. The truth probably lies somewhere in between, but given the lack of any other information and without the benefit of modern medical evidence, it is impossible at this point to ascertain just how ill he may have been after the war and whether and to what extent his military service affected his health.

Epilogue

After her husband's funeral, Eliza (McPherson) Underhill returned to Cambridge, Ohio, living at her parents' house with her three surviving children, Whittington, Nelle, and Eliza. For several years, life was uneventful, the children attending school and moving between the McPhersons' farm and their Cambridge house, depending on the season. Nelle said that she used to love to take a book and an apple, climb up into a tree and read. Her mother went back occasionally to Cincinnati, sometimes with the children, to visit with the Dunhams and to attend to estate matters. During this time there was a private girls' school in Cambridge, and Nelle recalled with amusement that it was common knowledge that later U.S. President William McKinley "was sweet on the headmistress."

Starting in November 1893, however, the family was to suffer three deaths in just over two years. On Sunday the 12th, Mrs. McPherson died rather suddenly at age seventy after a week's illness, leaving her husband bereft. Their daughters Mary Dunham and Jennie Ogier were financially secure, but Eliza Underhill and her three children were not. By early 1894, Dr. McPherson was almost seventy and in frail health, and by this time, Eliza Underhill and her family may have been aware that she was terminally ill. On February 12, 1894, McPherson deeded the farm to his three daughters, and on August 27, he and the Ogiers and the Dunhams deeded their interest in the Cambridge house to Eliza Underhill for one dollar.

A few days later, on September 3, 1894, Eliza Underhill, her family at

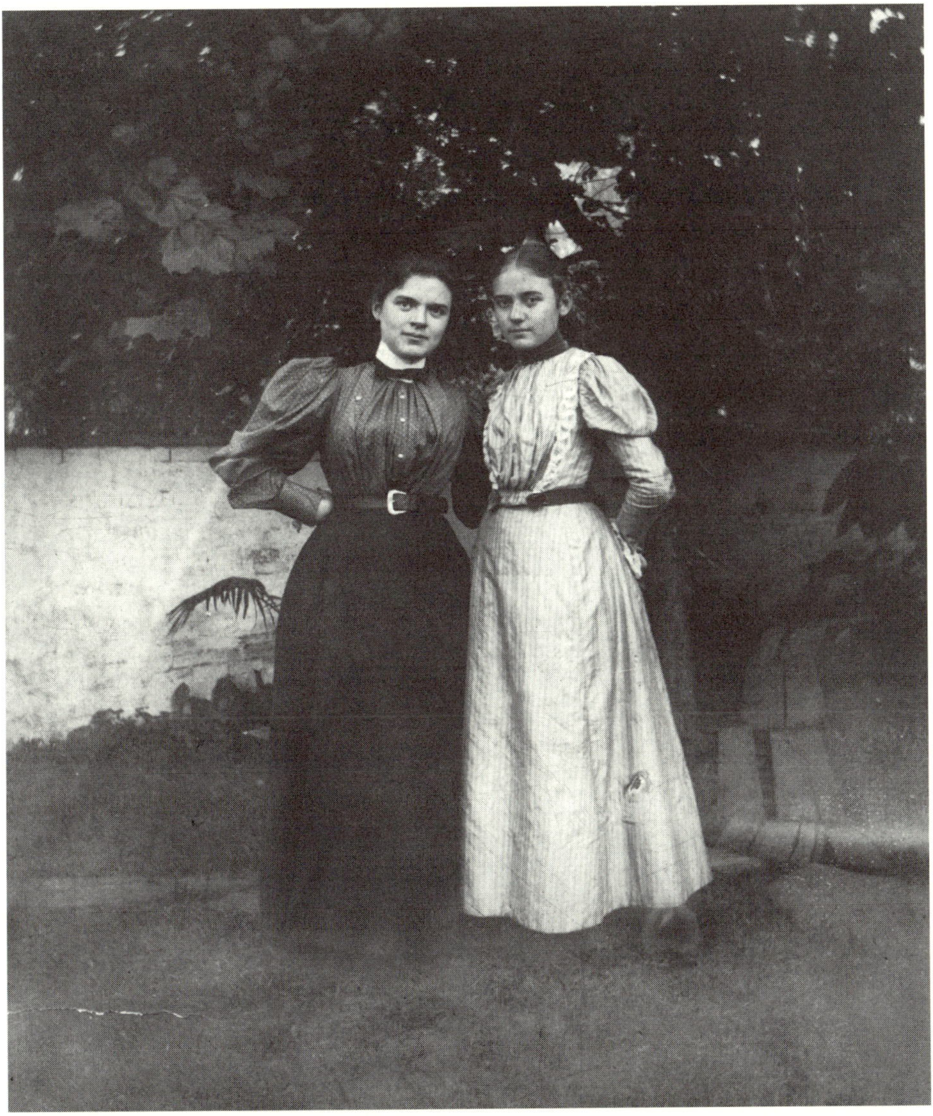

Already orphaned for three years, Joshua and Eliza (McPherson) Underhill's two surviving daughters, Nelle Abbot Underhill, 18, and Eliza Gilliland Underhill, 14, posed for this picture taken in Cincinnati on September 4, 1897. Eliza years later wrote on the back of the picture: "Us 'Glamorous'? Underhill girls!"

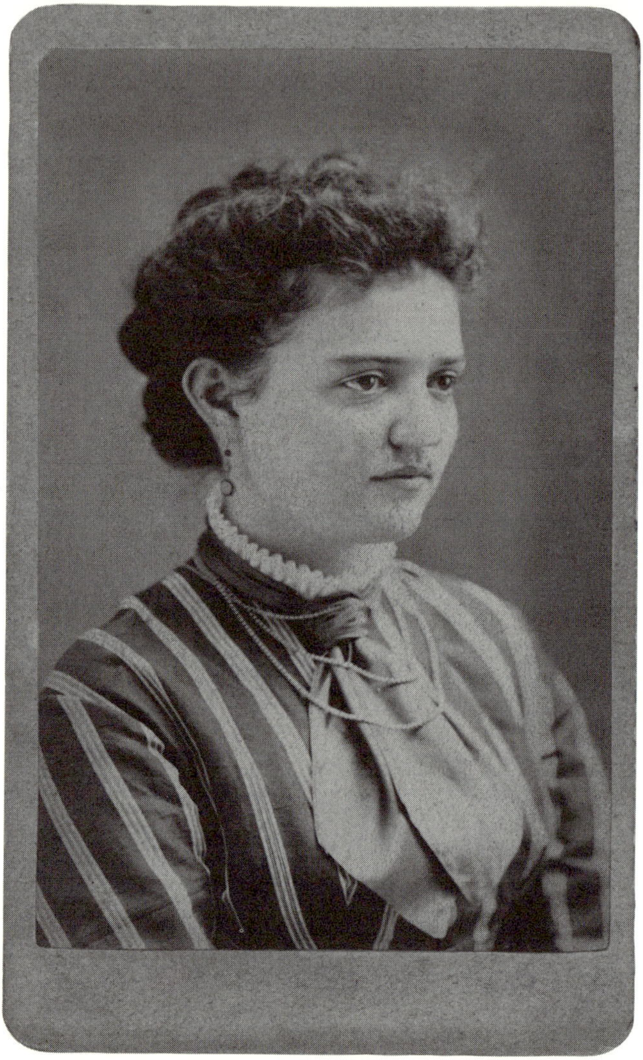

Jennie Crew (McPherson) Ogier (1857-1897), the youngest of the three McPherson sisters, married John M. Ogier and remained in Cambridge, Ohio. Although the Ogiers had no children, John Ogier became guardian of the Underhill children after Eliza (McPherson) Underhill died in 1894. This photograph of Jennie was taken about 1873.

her bedside, died after a long and painful struggle with rectal cancer at home in Cambridge, leaving Whittington, Nelle, and Eliza orphans. She was forty-five. After a funeral service at the house the next day, she was taken to Cincinnati and on September 5, interred in late afternoon beside her husband at Spring Grove. Her sisters, Mary Dunham and Jennie Ogier, became her joint executors, and John Ogier, Jennie's husband, became guardian of the children.

That school year, almost immediately after her mother's funeral, Nelle Underhill, by then fifteen, was sent to boarding school at the Swarthmore Grammar School, in Swarthmore, Pennsylvania, which she attended for two years. She was warm and welcoming and drew others to her, making good friends. She had happy memories of the school, ice skating along a frozen creek and pausing by its side to get hot chocolate, and on a couple of occasions, enjoying visits from slightly older Underhill second cousins, Albert and Harry, whose father, Joshua J. Underhill, had moved from Somerset County to Baltimore. Friends filled her autograph book with their addresses and morally uplifting sentiments. When Nelle went to boarding school at Swarthmore, her sister, Eliza, then eleven, was taken in by the Ogiers, who had no children of their own. No record remains of what Whittington was doing during this time.

Just before Nelle returned for Christmas vacation and only three months after her mother's death, Dr. McPherson caught influenza, which he was too weak to withstand, and late in the afternoon on December 15, 1894, he died peacefully at home. It had not occurred to Nelle when she left for school that she was seeing her grandfather for the last time. He died intestate, and David C. Kennon, a cousin and an attorney, became administrator of his now meager estate.

Nelle remembered her McPherson grandparents only in their later years. Although Dr. McPherson seems to have been kindly, she recalled that as a young girl, "I didn't like to kiss Grandfather, because he had a beard." Perhaps a careworn Mrs. McPherson might be forgiven peremptory treatment of her grandchildren – no doubt accommodating her widowed daughter and three grandchildren despite having a large house must have been difficult – but her granddaughter recalled her as a woman who brooked no nonsense and who must have been rather humorless. On one occasion, when the circus was coming to Cambridge, an event the children were eagerly anticipating, she made them go instead to the farm to help get animals under cover because of an impending storm. Nelle was a loving and gracious lady who never said anything unkind about her grandmother, but one could infer that quite unlike her adoration for her mother, she recalled Mary McPherson without much affection or sentimentality.

In 1897, another death occurred within the immediate family. Early in 1896, Jennie Ogier had contracted a serious illness – whose nature it has not been possible to ascertain – from which she seemed to have recovered, but it recurred, and in December, she and John had gone to stay with the Dunhams in Cincinnati to consult doctors there. However, nothing could be done, and Jennie died at 114 Dayton Street on January 2. She was only thirty-nine, and someone with a happy and sunny personality. John Ogier took her remains back to Cambridge, where the longtime pastor of the Presbyterian church, the Reverend Dr. William V. Milligan, who had buried her parents, conducted a funeral service at the Wheeling Avenue house, after which she was buried next to her parents in the City Cemetery in Cambridge. After Jennie's death, the Underhill children went to live with "Auntie Dunham," their sole surviving aunt, in Cincinnati in the Dayton Street house. Dr. Dunham's granddaughter, Mary McPherson Matthews Shuff, recalled her grandfather as "rather opinionated" – his was the day of the family patriarch – but remembered her grandmother as loving and kind. John Ogier remained in Cambridge where he died of typhoid fever in 1905 and was buried beside his wife.

By 1900, Cincinnati's West End had entered a decline. Its location in the river basin made it hot, and with all the industry, the air was not fresh. People lived there because they had to be close to their work. Lower class people were increasingly crowding into the tenements, and

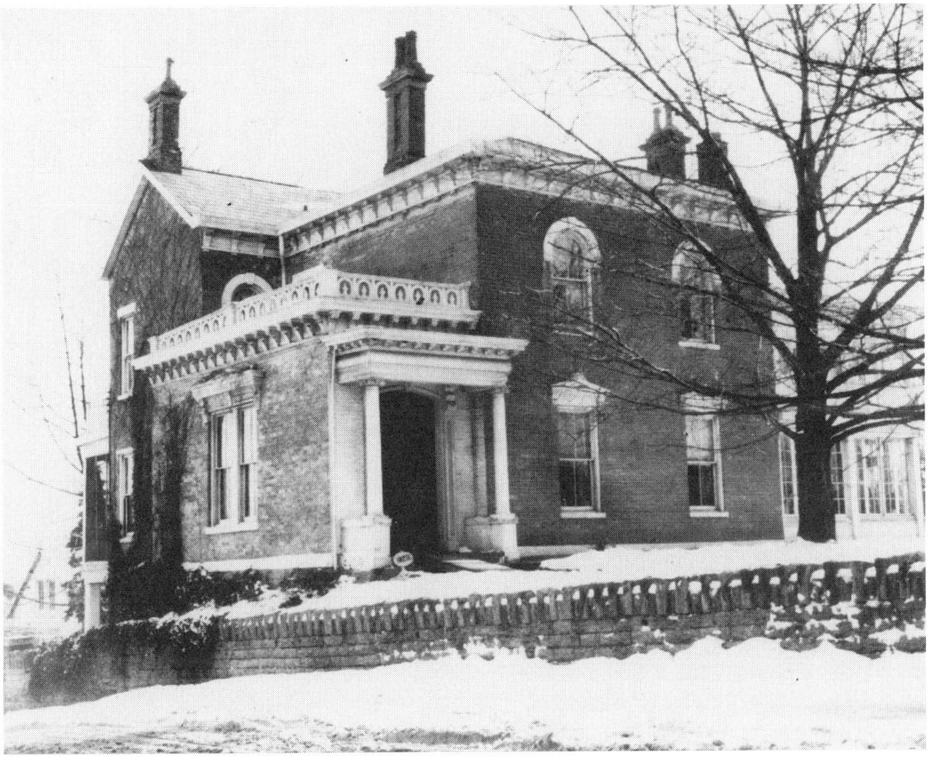

An Italianate-style house at 2340 Auburn Avenue in Cincinnati was acquired by Dr. William H. and Mary (McPherson) Dunham between 1900 and 1906. They both lived here for the remainder of their lives. Their daughter and son-in-law, Lida (Dunham) Matthews and Elijah H. Matthews, also lived with them. Another daughter and son-in-law, Mary (Dunham) Matthews and Judge Stanley Matthews, eventually took over the house. Not long after Judge Matthews died in 1963, the house was torn down for a medical building.

by this time, advancing technology brought streetcars which could ascend the steep Cincinnati hills, permitting people to live there but to get downtown easily. Mt. Auburn was one of the first hill suburbs to develop. At first, wealthier people had built there, but by the end of the century, the middle class was moving up as well. In 1899, the Dunhams sold the Dayton Street house for $14,000, $1000 less than they had paid for it, and moved up to rented quarters in an apartment block at 2509 Auburn Avenue, at the corner of McMillan Street. By this time, Kennon Dunham was in practice with his father, and for the first time, the office had a telephone. By 1906, the senior Dunhams were living a block away in a commodious house which they had bought at 2340 Auburn Avenue.

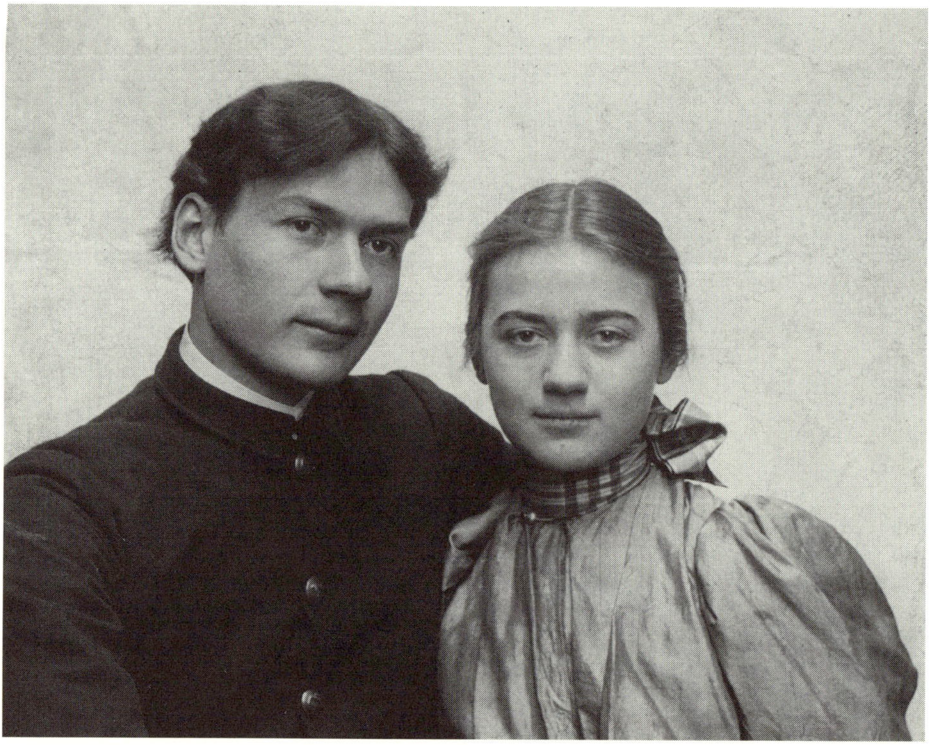

Whittington Townsend Underhill (1876-1903), the only son of Joshua and Eliza (McPherson) Underhill, posed with the younger of his sisters, Eliza Gilliland Underhill (1883-1970). Whittington would marry but not have children. His sister, Eliza, married Alexander Neil Flora. They had two children, Jane and Samuel Flora.

In 1900, Whittington Underhill completed law school at the University of Cincinnati and started a law partnership with Stanley Matthews, a law school classmate from New Vienna, Ohio. During their law school days, Stanley, at Whittington's invitation, had become a frequent visitor at Dayton Street, especially after meeting Whittington's cousin, Mary Dunham, and he continued to call on her after her parents moved to Mount Auburn. Stanley and Mary were married in October 1903, eventually having five children. In 1913, Stanley's brother Elijah married Mary's sister, Lida.

Shortly after finishing law school, Whittington had met and married Fanny Valentine Sloan, from Indiana. Nothing is known now of how they met, but they first lived in a house at 2114 Auburn Avenue, shortly moving to Rogers Place on Walnut Hills. In February 1903, the family suffered another terrible blow when Whittington contracted a virulent pneumonia that killed him in a week. He was twenty-six. Someone in the family recalled his wife nonchalantly munching on an apple at the door of the room where he lay dying, but neither Nelle nor Eliza ever recounted this story or ever spoke of Fanny, and what became of her is not known.

In 1904, Eliza Underhill had reached majority, and Mrs. Dunham, the remaining trustee of her sister's trust, deeded to Nelle and Eliza in equal shares the Cambridge house and the farm. The farm had been rented out, and in his guardianship report, John Ogier reported that after expenses, the farm was just breaking even. The same year, David C. Kennon closed out Dr. McPherson's estate, after selling the shares of Quaker State Bank stock remaining in it.

Nelle Underhill, after two years at Swarthmore and a job at the Treasury Department in Washington, returned to Cincinnati, living with the Dunhams and working as a clerk. On January 29, 1901 the Reverend Melville Curtis officiated at her wedding to Philip Hayward of Cincinnati. She was twenty-one, he was twenty-two. Philip had served in the Spanish-American War and had been a year ahead of Whittington Underhill and Stanley Matthews at law school. Philip was an only child whose father, Charles Hayward, had died of tuberculosis when Philip was six. His mother, Anna (Hurd) Hayward, then took him on an

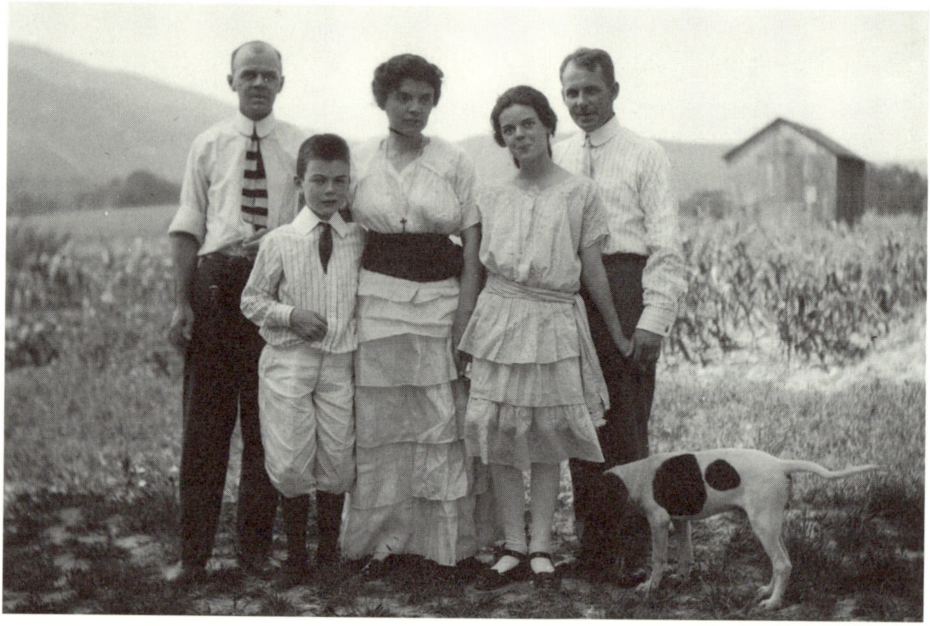

Nelle Underhill, the third child of Joshua and Eliza (McPherson) Underhill, was married twice, having two children by her first marriage. Gathered about her in this photograph taken about 1914 are (left to right): Nelle's first husband, Spanish-American War veteran Philip Hayward (1878-1931); their son and Joshua Underhill's grandson, Richard Folsom Hayward (1903-1981); Nelle (Underhill) Hayward (1879-1979); her daughter and Joshua Underhill's granddaughter, Marion Hayward (1902-1972); and George Gordon Green (c. 1878-1939), an army friend of Philip Hayward who would later become Nelle's second husband.

extended tour of Europe, after which she returned to Cincinnati and in 1896 married William W. Symmes. Philip and Nelle (Underhill) Hayward had two children, Marion (1902-1972) and Richard Folsom (1903-1981), but the marriage nearly ended several years later after Philip had a liaison with a secretary resulting in an illegitimate daughter. He eventually came back but disappeared in December 1914. Disgusted by his behavior, his family supported Nelle, and in 1919, she obtained a divorce after suing on the grounds of abandonment. In 1930 she married Gordon Green, an old friend who had been widowed, and they enjoyed a happy marriage until his untimely death in September 1939. She continued to live in Cincinnati in their apartment at 3021 Fairfield Avenue, where she died in January 1979 at age 99. Her ashes were placed in her beloved mother's grave.

Philip moved around, having little contact with his children. During World War I, he worked as an accountant at the Bremerton, Washington Navy Yard. In 1918 he was reported to be working on a ranch near Kemmerer, Wyoming, not in the best of health, and living with a woman he alleged to be his wife, whose maiden name was Lida Hayes. They did marry, but when has not been ascertained. In 1920 he moved to Watsonville, California, becoming deputy county clerk in Santa Cruz. In 1926 he became the first elected justice of the peace there. He was active in the local Spanish-American veterans post and a member of the Rotary club. He died in Watsonville in February 1931 after a year's illness with myocarditis.

Eliza Underhill married Alexander Neil Flora, who became a prominent steel executive. They lived first in Warren, Ohio where he was president of Trumble Steel and one of the original members of the American Flat-Rolled Steel Association, which later became the American Iron and Steel Institute. They later moved to Sewickley, Pennsylvania. After his death in 1942, she moved to California to join their two children, Jane (1905-1983) and Samuel (1907-1994), first living at Laguna Beach, then in Pasadena before moving in the early 1950s to a bungalow in LaJolla, where she remained until her death in 1970. Neil and Eliza (Underhill) Flora and their two children are buried at Oakwood Cemetery in Warren, Ohio.

Dr. and Mrs. Dunham remained at 2340 Auburn Avenue until their deaths in 1925 and 1931, respectively. A photograph of them taken late in life depicts a tall, bearded, white-haired gentleman of impassive demeanor beside a strong, wide-faced lady of great character whose burden as care giver for the whole family has left her with an expression of overwhelming weariness. After she died, her house was taken over by then Judge and Mrs. Stanley Matthews.

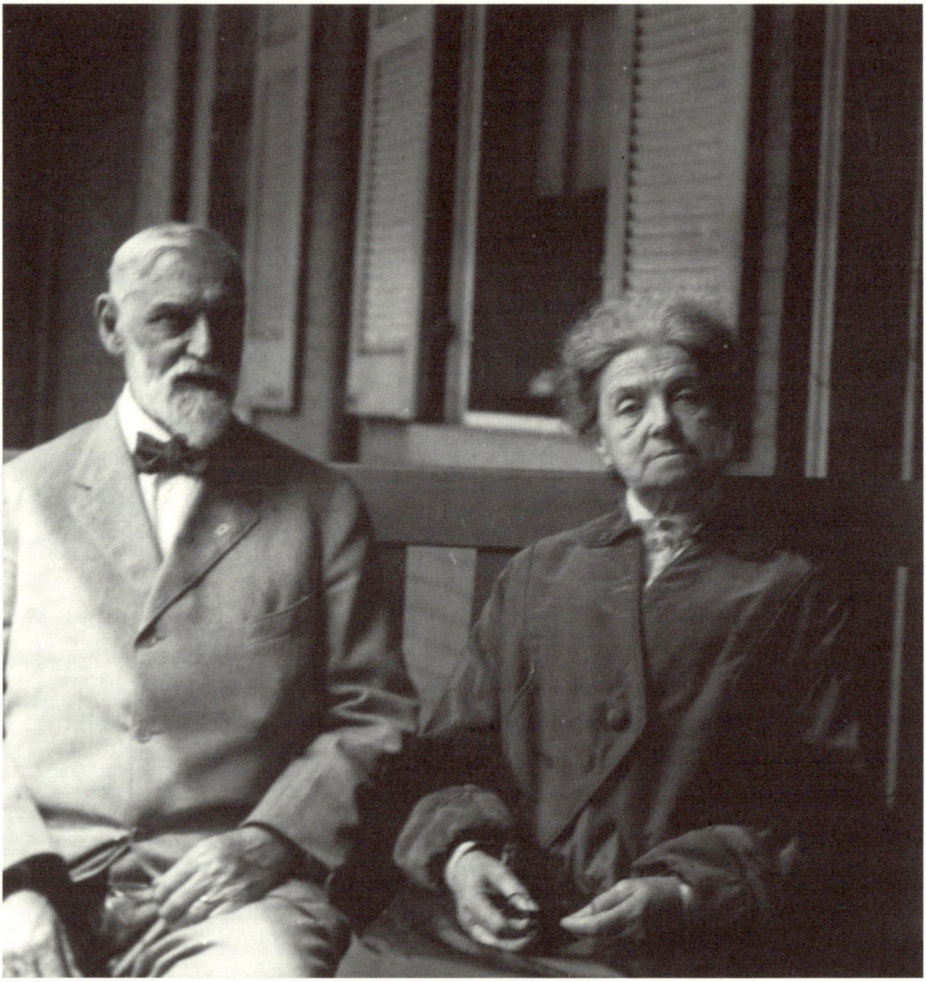

Living until 1931, Mary (McPherson) Dunham was the last survivor of the three McPherson sisters. The daughter of Dr. Jeremiah Townsend McPherson and the sister-in-law of Civil War diarist Joshua Whittington Underhill, she had herself married a doctor, William Henry Dunham, and their three children included a son who became a doctor. The Dunhams ultimately helped to raise the Underhill children in their Cincinnati home. Dr. and Mrs. Dunham sat for this photograph about 1918.

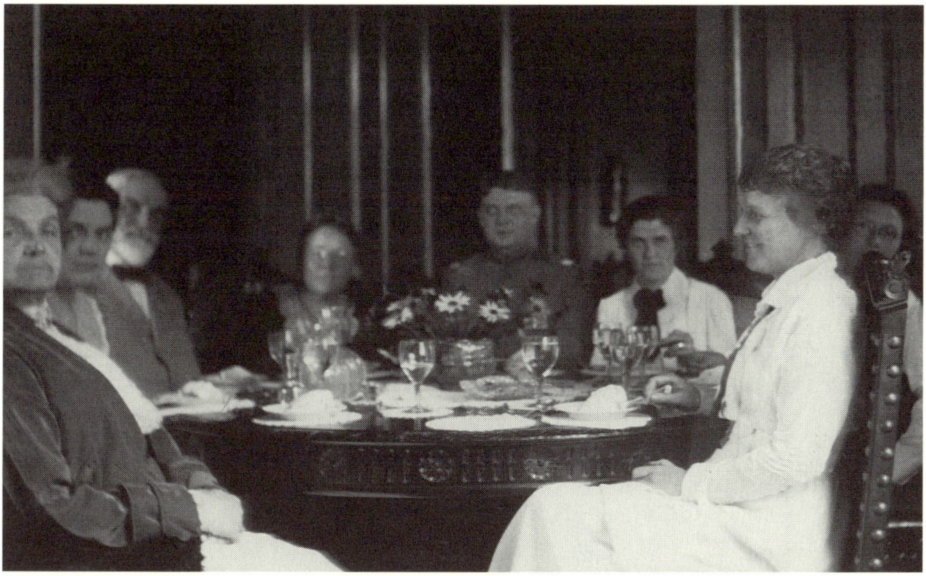

On what may have been Easter about 1918, family gathered around the table at Nelle (Underhill) Hayward's Cincinnati home at 2355 Auburn Avenue. Gathered (from left to right) were: Underhill's sister-in-law, Mary McPherson Dunham (1850-1931); Underhill's daughter, Nelle (Underhill) Hayward (1879-1979); Mary's husband, Dr. William Henry Dunham (1846-1925); their daughter-in-law, Amelia (Hickenlooper) Dunham (1874-1944): her husband, Dr. Henry Kennon Dunham (1872-1944), dressed in his military uniform of World War I; his sister, Lida (Dunham) Matthews (1881-1950), youngest of the three Dunham siblings; and behind an unknown lady dressed in white was their other sister, Mary (Dunham) Matthews (1878-1939).

The West End of Cincinnati has changed greatly since the Underhills and Dunhams lived there. The Dunham house at 428 Baymiller Street is gone. The houses along Dayton Street remain largely intact, but the neighborhood became terribly run down, and the Dunham house, now number 830 after the 1896 street renumbering, is divided into apartments. It looks neglected, but its grandeur remains. Historic preservation interests are gradually trying to restore the street. The houses on John and Clinton Streets that the Underhills lived in were all pulled down in 1954 to make room for playing fields for the new Taft High School. On Mt. Auburn, neither the apartment block at 2309 nor the house at 2340 Auburn Avenue still stands. Dr. McPherson's stone house in Cambridge is also gone.

At the top of a pretty slope overlooking a quiet reflecting pond in Spring Grove Cemetery, a Celtic cross with the names *Underhill, Dunham,* and *Matthews* engraved around its base stands where many of the family have almost filled the plot that Dr. Dunham and Mrs. Underhill bought over a hundred years ago.

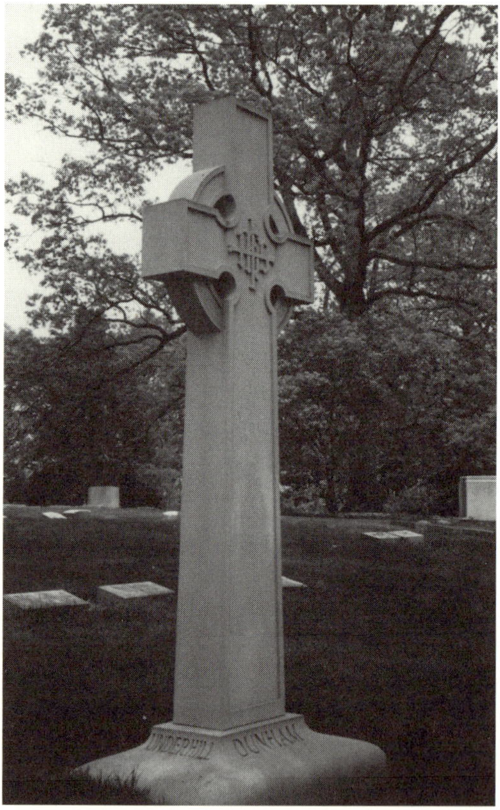

A Celtic cross marks the Underhill-Dunham-Matthews lot at Spring Grove Cemetery in Cincinnati.

Envoi

When Joshua Whittington Underhill died, Dr. Abijah J. Miles, his contemporary and a colleague at the Cincinnati College of Medicine and Surgery, commented that "His case was a sad one. He was a bright man and had a glorious future before him."

The American playwright Arthur Miller has observed that for an outcome to be not merely pathetic but tragic, we must have fear for what will happen to a character, and that a character must have "missed accomplishing his joy." Dead at only fifty-two but hopelessly in the claws of addiction for at least two years before that and thereby cut off from the glorious future that Dr. Miles envisioned, Underhill's end was indeed tragic.

Despite the tragedy surrounding his end, however, his achievements remain as testimony to a man who accomplished much in the time that he had. Even today, well over a century after his death, his work is remembered. In July 1998, Joshua Whittington Underhill was inducted into the *Cincinnati Medicine* Hall of Honor, the citation reading:

Joshua Whittington Underhill
(1837-1889)
Nationally acclaimed gynecologist,
pioneer of the specialty of Medical Jurisprudence.

End Notes

Origins

1 Edwin R. Deats, comp., *Underhill Genealogy* vol. VI Harry Macy, Jr., ed. (Baltimore: Gateway Press, Inc., 1980) 1302.

2 Deats 1313.

3 Otto Juettner, *Daniel Drake and His Followers* (Cincinnati: Harvey Publishing Company, 1909) 308.

4 Arthur G. King, *The Cincinnati Obstetrical and Gynecological Society 1876-1976* (Cincinnati: Merrell - National Laboratories, 1976) 26.

5 *Cincinnati Enquirer*, 29 Jan. 1889, 1.

6 Deats 1313.

7 William G. Wolfe *Stories of Guernsey County, Ohio*: History of an Average Ohio County Cambridge, Ohio: printed privately by the author, 1943) 953.

Background to the Conflict and The Early War Years

8 William T. Sherman *Memoirs of General William T. Sherman* (New York: D. Appleton and Company, 1886) vol. I, 177, 178.

9 Sherman 181.

10 W. H. Hamelle *A Standard History of White County, Indiana* (Chicago and New York: The Lewis Publishing Company, 1915) vol. I, 179, 180.

11 Hamelle 180.

12 Hamelle 181.

13 Thomas H. Bringhurst and Frank Swigart, compilers, *History of the Forty-Sixth Regiment Indiana Volunteer Infantry* (Logansport, Indiana: Wilson, Humphreys & Co., 1888), 12.

14 Bringhurst and Swigart 30.

Helena

15 Sherman 308.

16 U.S. Grant *Personal Memoirs of U.S. Grant* (New York: Charles L. Webster & Company, 1885) vol. I 449, 450.

Vicksburg

17 Grant 463.

18 Grant 474 - 476.

19 Grant 493, 494.

20 Emma Balfour, *Diary of Emma Balfour, May 16, 1863 - June 2, 1863*, copyright 1983, Phillip C. Weinberger.

21 Sherman 324, 325

22 Grant 440, 441.

23 Sherman 330, 331.

24 Grant 546, 547.

25 Sherman 359.

After Vicksburg

26 Bringhurst and Swigart 96.

27 *Report of W.H.H. Terrell, Adjutant General, Indiana, 1861-1865* (Indianapolis: W. R. Holloway, State Publisher, 1865) vol. II, 461, 462.

28 Bringhurst and Swigart 116.

Life After the War

29 King 22.
30 King 25. (The article was included in: *The American Journal of Obstetrics*, Vol. XII, No.1, 1879, 91-111.)
31 King 26-28.

The Final Period

32 *Cincinnati Enquirer,* 29 Jan. 1889, 1.
33 Cincinnati Enquirer, 30 Jan. 1889, 5.
34 *Enquirer*, 1.
35 *Enquirer*, 5.
36 King, 28·

Selected Bibliography

Ambrose, Stephen E. *Struggle for Vicksburg*. Eastern Acorn Press, 1992.

Atkinson, Willliam B., ed. *Physicians and Surgeons of the United States.* Philadelphia: Charles Robson, 1878.

Balfour, Emma. *Diary of Emma Balfour, May 16, 1863 - June 2, 1863.* Copyright 1983 by Phillip C. Weinberger.

Bringhurst, Thomas H. and Frank Swigart, comps. *History of the Forty-Sixth Indiana Volunteer Infantry.* Logansport, Indiana: Wilson, Humphreys & Co., 1888.

Caldwell, J. A. *History of Belmont and Jefferson Counties, Ohio.* Wheeling, West Virginia: The Historical Publishing Company, 1880.

Craik, Dinah Maria Mulock. *John Halifax Gentleman.* New York: Harper & Brothers, 1903.

Davis, William C. and Bell I. Wiley, eds. *Photographic History of the Civil War: Fort Sumter to Gettysburg*. New York: Black Dog & Leventhan Publishers, 1994.

Deats, Edwin R., comp. *Underhill Genealogy.* 6 vols. Harry Macy, Jr., ed. Baltimore: Gateway Press, Inc. 1980.

de Man, George E. N., comp. and ed. *Helena: The Ridge, The River, The Romance.* Little Rock, Arkansas: Pioneer Press, 1978.

Fox, Jim. *Where We Live.* St. Louis: Missouri Historical Society Press, 1995.

Goodrich, DeWitt C. and Charles R. Tuttle. *An Illustrated History of the State of Indiana.* Indianapolis: Richard S. Peake & Co., Publisher, 1875.

Grant, U.S. *Personal Memoirs of U.S. Grant. Vol. I.* New York: Charles L. Webster & Company, 1885.

Guernsey, Alfred H. and Henry M. Alden. *Harper's Pictorial History of the Civil War.* Avenel, New Jersey: Gramercy Books, originally published in 1866.

Hamelle, W. H. *A Standard History of White County Indiana.* Chicago and New York: The Lewis Publishing Company, 1915.

The History of Brown County, Ohio. Chicago: W. H. Beers & Co., 1883. Reprinted by Higginson Book Company, Salem, Massachusetts.

Hoehling, A. A. *Vicksburg 47 Days of Siege.* Mechanicsburg, Pennsylvania: Stackpole Books, 1996.

Indiana. Adjutant General's Office. *Report of W. H. H. Terrell, Adjutant General, Indiana 1861-1865.* Indianapolis: W. R. Holloway, State Publisher, 1865.

Iowa. Adjutant General's Office. *Report of Brig. Gen. Nathaniel B. Baker, Adjutant General and Acting Q. M. G. and acting as P. M.*

G. to the Governor of the State of Iowa. Des Moines: F. W. Palmer, State Printer, 1867.

Juettner, Otto. *Daniel Drake and His Followers.* Cincinnati: Harvey Publishing Company, 1909.

King, Arthur G. *The Cincinnati Obstetrical and Gynecological Society 1876-1976.* Cincinnati: Merrell-National Laboratories, 1976.

McKelvey, A.T., comp. and ed. *Centennial History of Belmont County, Ohio and Representative Citizens.* Chicago, Illinois: Biographical Publishing Co., 1903.

McPherson, James M. *Battle Cry of Freedom.* New York: Ballantine Books, 1988.

Missouri. Adjutant General's Office. *Report of the Adjutant General of Missouri.* Jefferson City: W. A. Curry, Public Printer, 1864.

Rutkow, Ira M. *An Alphabetical List of the Battles of the War of the Rebellion and a Roster of all the Regimental Surgeons and Assistant Surgeons.* San Francisco: Norman Publishing, 1990.

Sherman, William T. *Memoirs of General William T. Sherman.* Vol I. New York: D. Appleton and Company, 1886.

Sifakis, Stewart. *Who Was Who in the Civil War.* New York: Facts on File, Inc., 1988.

Warner, Susan. *The Hills of the Shatemuc.* New York: D. Appleton and Company, 1856.

Way, Frederick Jr., comp. *Way's Packet Directory 1848-1994.* Athens: Ohio University Press, 1994.

Wilson, Woodrow T. *Thirty-Four Families of Old Somerset County, Maryland.* Baltimore, Maryland: Gateway Press, Inc., 1974.

Wisconsin. Adjutant General's Office. *Annual Report of the Adjutant General of the State of Wisconsin with Reports from the Quartermaster General and Surgeon General for the year ending December 31, 1864.* Madison, Wisconsin: Atwood & Rublee, State Printers, 1865.

Wise, Matthew M. *The Littleton Heritage.* West Columbia, South Carolina: The Wentworth Publishing Corporation, 1997.

Wolfe, William G. *Stories of Guernsey County, Ohio: History of an Average Ohio County.* Cambridge, Ohio: privately printed by the author, 1943.

Chronology

1837 Joshua Whittington Underhill is born January 11 in Quindocqua, Somerset County, Maryland, to Thomas Henry and Eleanor (Whittington) Underhill.

1840 Underhill's mother dies after childbirth in Belmont County, Ohio, while the family is en route to Missouri. The infant dies and Underhill's father leaves, not to be heard from again. Underhill is taken in by John and Eleanor (McPherson) Gilbert of Hendrysburg, later of Fairview, Ohio. They become "home" and he will be shown on the census with them by name in 1850 and 1860.

1856 Underhill begins the first of two years at Madison College in Antrim, Guernsey County, Ohio.

1858 Underhill begins studying medicine with Dr. Jeremiah T. McPherson in Fairview, Guernsey County, Ohio.

1860 Underhill goes to Cincinnati to complete his medical training at the Cincinnati College of Medicine and Surgery.

1861 On April 12, the first hostilities of the Civil War break out when Confederates fire upon Fort Sumter in Charleston, South Carolina. Underhill completes his medical degree requirements but is not officially awarded the degree until 1865. After a visit to his home in Fairview, Ohio he sets off in mid-July for Burnettsville, White County, Indiana, to begin practicing medicine. On October 13, he enlists as a Private in Company E, 46th Regiment, Indiana Volunteer Infantry, and reports to Camp Logan, Logansport, Indiana. He almost immediately becomes a Hospital Steward. On December 12, Underhill's regiment is mustered into service and departs Logansport. By Christmas, the regiment is in Bardstown, Kentucky.

1862 Underhill's regiment arrives at Camp Wickliffe, Kentucky, on January 7, remaining until February 14. Underhill, left behind in charge of the sick, leaves three days later in search of his unit, to find it a month later at New Madrid, Missouri.

After the victory at New Madrid, the 46th moves south to Riddle's Point, and constructs a battery on the Mississippi River on March 18-19. On April 9, the regiment crosses to Tiptonville, Tennessee, leaving April 13 under General Pope for Fort Pillow. On April 16, they arrive at Osceola, Arkansas, but the next day, General Halleck recalls most of the forces to Shiloh. Underhill's unit stays at Osceola until Fort Pillow is evacuated on June 4. Underhill is very ill with malaria and jaundice during this time. On June 6 the Indiana 43rd and 46th take control of Memphis, remaining until June 15. The 46th then goes on an expedition up the White River in Arkansas to rendezvous with forces of General Samuel Curtis and gets into a fight at St. Charles, Arkansas, on June 17. In mid-July Underhill's regiment arrives at Helena, Arkansas, where, in October, Underhill buys his diary and makes his first entry on October 23. On November 16 he documents the start of an abortive attempt to take Arkansas Post and on December 7 the results of a more successful raid into Mississippi, although he merely observes from Helena. On December 21, Underhill watches troops head down river on the ill-fated Chickasaw Bayou assault of December 29. His diary entry on New Year's Eve reflects the terrible tragedy of the war.

1863 On January 10 Underhill receives his commission as Assistant Surgeon, dating from December 30. From January 11–21, Underhill goes on another expedition up the White River, returning to Helena January 23. On February 15 the 46th leaves on the first Yazoo Pass expedition and after only one day in Helena, departs again February 24 on the second expedition. Underhill remains in Helena. The regiment returns April 9. Underhill leaves Helena April 11 with his regiment for Milliken's Bend, Louisiana on the start of the Vicksburg Campaign. On April 16 Underhill leaves Milliken's Bend. The Indiana 46th is among the first units to cross to Bruinsburg, Mississippi on April 30. It fights in the Battle of Port Gibson on May 1, then moves northeast towards Jackson, Mississippi. On May 16, Underhill witnesses the Battle of Champion Hill. By May 25 the 46th is at Vicksburg, where it remains until the siege ends on July 4. July 6 Underhill marches east towards Jackson and is overcome by heatstroke. On July 16 Jackson is evacuated and on July 21, Underhill's unit leaves for Vicksburg. He loses his diary that night and when he realizes it the next day, he is too far away to return for it. The regiment reaches Vicksburg July 23 and stays until August 4, when it goes to Natchez, where Underhill has another malaria attack. Underhill's jockeying with Israel Washburn for promotion to regimental Surgeon starts at this time. The 46th leaves Natchez August 15 for Carrollton, Louisiana, remaining for three weeks. From September to December, the regiment operates in southwestern Louisiana but for November and December, Underhill is on detached duty in charge of the hospital at New Iberia.

1864 On January 2 Underhill reenlists as a veteran. The 46th is at Algiers, Louisiana until January 19, when it moves across Lake Ponchartrain to Madisonville, returning on February 27. On March 4 Underhill's regiment moves with General Banks on the disastrous Red River Campaign, suffering severe losses and not returning to New Orleans until late May. On June 12 the regiment departs for Logansport for much deserved furlough, reassembling there on July 26. The regiment is sent on various expeditions in Kentucky and Virginia. Anticipating the departure of regimental Surgeon Israel Washburn in December, Colonel Bringhurst of the 46th writes Indiana Governor Morton on August 6 endorsing Underhill's promotion to Surgeon. The year's end finds Underhill in Lexington, Kentucky.

1865 On January 12 Underhill writes directly to Governor Morton, asking about the post of regimental Surgeon. A letter from Colonel Bringhurst written January 19 brings no reply, and on January 30, Underhill writes Governor Morton again. On February 6 Underhill gets his promotion to Surgeon, to date from January 1. Until June Underhill serves as Post Surgeon at prisons 3 and 4 in Lexington, Kentucky. He then transfers to Louisville, Kentucky, where he remains until mustered out with the regiment on September 4. He then goes to New York, taking up study at the Bellevue Hospital Medical College.

1866 Underhill leaves Bellevue in May and settles in Cincinnati, opening an office with George K. Taylor. In September he joins the faculty at the Cincinnati College of Medicine and Surgery as a demonstrator of anatomy.

1869 Underhill and Taylor end their joint practice.

1870 Underhill is elected Coroner for Hamilton County and is away from his teaching duties for two years. He becomes an expert on medical jurisprudence.

1872 Underhill returns to the Cincinnati College of Medicine and Surgery as a lecturer in medical jurisprudence, a post he holds for seven years.

1873 Underhill's Civil War diary is returned to him in November by C. G. Jennings of Delaware, Ohio.

1874 In June, Underhill marries Eliza McPherson, the eldest daughter of Jeremiah T. McPherson, his medical preceptor, in Fairview, Ohio, and brings his bride to live at 434 John Street in Cincinnati.

1875 The Underhills' first child, Mary Eleanor, is born on August 4.

1876 Underhill joins with eleven others to found the Cincinnati Obstetrical Society. He is elected to the Cincinnati School Board. In October the Underhills buy a house at 418 John Street in Cincinnati, although they do not occupy it. On December 29, their only son, Whittington Townsend Underhill, is born.

1877 Underhill becomes the first secretary of the Cincinnati Obstetrical Society, a post he will hold for two years.

1878 Underhill is reelected to the Cincinnati School Board. In November he gives a paper to the Cincinnati Obstetrical Society entitled " The Female Generative Organs in their Medico-Legal Relations," which becomes a classic in medical jurisprudence.

1879 Underhill becomes professor of Materia Medica at the Cincinnati College of Medicine and Surgery. He also becomes the second president of the Cincinnati Obstetrical Society. On July 28 the Underhills' third child, Nelle Abbot, is born.

1880 Underhill becomes a professor of Obstetrics, a post he will hold for two years. He signs a five-year lease on a house at 26 Clinton Street. Underhill becomes president of Cincinnati School Board for two years and serves on the Board of Examiners for teachers.

1881 Mary Eleanor Underhill dies on April 15, shortly before her sixth birthday. This is a crushing blow for Underhill.

1882 On February 25, the Underhill's fourth child, Jean, is born. She dies on November 1. Underhill does not return to the Cincinnati College of Medicine and Surgery in the fall. He goes into practice with William H. Dunham, his wife's brother-in-law.

1884 According to one account, Underhill begins experimenting with cocaine.

1885 In August, the Underhills take out a mortgage on the John Street property which will be foreclosed after his death in 1889.

1886 Underhill's partner, William H. Dunham, withdraws from their partnership. Underhill is addicted to cocaine by this time and cannot practice. He becomes paranoid and suffers hallucinations. Eliza Underhill leaves him and goes with the three surviving children to live with her parents in Cambridge, Ohio.

1887 In May Underhill files for an invalid pension. In September the Adjutant General's Office informs the Commissioner of Pensions that records indicate no evidence of disability as an enlisted man. In December a similar report finds no disability as an officer. Underhill does not pursue the claim.

1888 Underhill's colleague Thaddeus Reamy sees Underhill for the last time and recognizes that nothing can be done. In the spring, another colleague, Dr. Wenning, without success urges Underhill to go into a sanitarium.

1889 Underhill dies at home at noon on Monday, January 28, of tetanus. A rusted fork dropping on an ankle and puncturing it is alleged to be the cause. Eliza Underhill comes from Cambridge the next day. His funeral is held at Spring Grove Cemetery on Wednesday, January 30, and he is buried in a lot owned by Mary McMurphy next to his daughters Mary Eleanor and Jean.

1893 Underhill with his daughters Mary Eleanor and Jean are moved to their final resting places in Spring Grove Cemetery.

Descendants of Joshua W. & Eliza (McPherson) Underhill

1 Joshua Whittington Underhill 1837 - 1889
+Eliza McPherson 1849 - 1894
2 Mary Eleanor Underhill 1875 - 1881
2 Whittington Townsend Underhill 1876 - 1903
+Fanny Valentine Sloan
2 Nelle Abbot Underhill 1879 - 1979
+Philip Hayward 1878 - 1931
3 Marion Hayward 1902 - 1972
+William Power Clancey 1895 - 1984
4 Anna Hurd Clancey 1925 -
+Walter Higbee Caskey 1921 -
5 Alexander Floyd Caskey 1946 -
+Clara Angelica de Oliveira Porto 1949 -
6 Sasha Porto Caskey 1974 -
+Marina Fernandes de Barros 1974 -
6 Vanessa Porto Caskey 1976 -
*2nd Wife of Alexander Floyd Caskey:
+Maria del Carmen Lozano Velasco 1945 -
5 Noelle Caskey 1947 -
+Richard Freudenheim 1946 -
5 Jennifer Hurd Caskey 1950 -
+Steven Patrick Kelleher 1949 -
*2nd Husband of Jennifer Hurd Caskey:
+John Frederic Kolhouse 1943 -
5 Nicholas Hayward Caskey 1952 -
+Susan Sachiko Nakamura 1957 -
4 William Power Clancey, Jr. 1926 -
+Barbara Ann Hopper 1930 -
5 Timothy Logan Clancey 1950 -
+Mary Lou Meyer 1954 - 1978
*2nd Wife of Timothy Logan Clancey:
+Jean Brown 1945 -
6 Lauren Forrester Clancey 1980 -
6 Joel William Clancey 1983 -
6 Patrick Timothy Clancey 1983 -
5 Colleen Anne Clancey 1952 -
+Michael Anderson
*2nd Husband of Colleen Anne Clancey:
+Joshua Brown 1953 -
5 Eileen Siobhan Clancey 1953 -
+Kevin DeCoster 1953 -
6 Brendan James DeCoster 1981 -
6 Cameron Daniel Clancey DeCoster 1983 -
*2nd Husband of Eileen Siobhan Clancey:
+Thomas Gerald Burns 1953 -
6 Connor Thomas Clancey - Burns 1993 -
5 William Power Clancey III 1954 -
+Margaret Knifton 1947 -
6 Christopher Ryan Clancey 1990 -
*2nd Wife of William Power Clancey, Jr.:
+Patricia Pace 1929 -
4 Richard Folsom Hayward Clancey 1928 -
+Marion Cole 1928 -
5 Laurence Hayward Clancey 1955 -
+Susan Nelson 1955 -
6 Andrew Nelson Clancey 1984 -
6 Peter Laurence Clancey 1989 -
5 Cole Mann Clancey 1957 -
*2nd Husband of Marion Hayward:
+Noel Morss 1904 - 1981
4 Christopher Morss 1940 -

3 Richard Folsom Hayward 1903 - 1981
+Ruth Morison Faulkner 1897 - 1973
4 Ellen Hayward 1935 - 1989
+Charles Roentsch 1934 - 1983
5 Peter Roentsch 1957 -
+Amelia Carignan 1964 -
6 Alison Amelia Roentsch 1987 -
6 Jennifer Ellen Roentsch 1990 -
*2nd Wife of Peter Roentsch:
+Cathy Lorette 1960 -
*2nd Husband of Ellen Hayward:
+Martin Walsh
4 James Duncan Hurd Hayward 1937 -
4 Timothy Yeatman Hayward 1941 -
+Susan Howard Cady 1948 -
5 Heidi Arnold Hayward 1969 -
+Steven Joseph Urish 1970 -
6 Emily Morison Hayward Urish 1999 -
5 Nathaniel Morison Hayward 1972 -
5 Zachary Cady Hayward 1978 -
*2nd Wife of Richard Folsom Hayward:
+Mary Hart 1914 - 1985
4 Richard Folsom Hayward, Jr. 1947 -
+Vivian Marina Valdes 1950 -
5 Yvette Lyn Hayward 1974 -
+Gustavo Angel Velasquez 1973
6 Tatianna Velasquez 1994 -
4 Philip Carey Hayward 1949 -
+Pauline Marie Lange 1947 -
5 Clara Hart Hayward 1986 -
4 Geoffrey Hart Hayward 1950 - 1987
4 Jonathan Underhill Hayward 1956 -
+Leslie Ann Carter 1957 -
*2nd Wife of Jonathan Underhill Hayward:
+Kimberlee Anne Morton 1961 -
4 Alexander Duncan Hayward 1959 -
*2nd Husband of Nelle Abbot Underhill:
+George Gordon Green abt 1878 - 1939
2 Jean Underhill 1882 - 1882
2 Eliza Gilliland Underhill 1883 - 1970
+Alexander Neil Flora 1878 - 1942
3 Jane Flora 1905 - 1983
+James W. Hume, Jr. 1901 - 1931
*2nd Husband of Jane Flora:
+Marcel Petit
*3rd Husband of Jane Flora:
+James Ware abt 1915 -
3 Samuel Bennett Flora 1907 - 1994
+Dorothy Corbett 1911 - 1978
4 Alexander Neil Flora 1934 -
+Evanne Leland
*2nd Wife of Alexander Neil Flora:
+Norma Salem
5 Jennifer Anne Flora 1973 -
*3rd Wife of Alexander Neil Flora:
+Kathy Richter 1947 -
4 Samuel Bennett Flora, Jr. 1936 -
+Anne Marie Noid 1938 -
5 Elizabeth Anne Flora 1968 -
5 Corbett Patrick Flora 1972 -

Descendants of William H. & Mary (McPherson) Dunham

1 William Henry Dunham 1846 - 1925
+Mary Kennon McPherson 1850 - 1931
2 Henry Kennon Dunham 1872 - 1944
+Amelia Hickenlooper 1874 - 1946
3 Amelia Kennon Dunham 1906 - 1989
3 Harry Hickenlooper Dunham 1910 - 1944
2 Mary Letitia Dunham 1878 - 1939
+Stanley Matthews 1878 - 1963
3 Mary McPherson Matthews 1904 - 1997
+Thomas Kilby Shuff 1900 - 1973
4 Thomas Kilby Shuff, Jr. 1934 -
+Janice Sue Gierman 1938 -
5 Thomas Kilby Shuff IV 1958 -
+Jennifer Louise Cobb abt 1960 -
*2nd Wife of Thomas Kilby Shuff IV:
+Rayanne Michie Mori 1958 -
*3rd Wife of Thomas Kilby Shuff IV:
+Lana Kay Tanaka 1970 -
5 Matthew Layton Shuff 1959 -
+Denise Sisk 1959 -
6 Craig Allen Shuff 1981 -
6 Stephanie Dyan Shuff 1983 -
6 Eric Layton Shuff 1985 -
5 Susan Davidson Shuff 1961 -
+Christopher Lynn McCabe 1958 -
*2nd Husband of Susan Davidson Shuff:
+Thomas James Burger 1960 -
6 Mary McPherson Burger 1993 -
6 Mark Thomas Burger 1997 -
6 Anna Davidson Burger 1999 -
5 Karen Lynne Shuff 1963 -
+Stirling Earl Farris Sampson 1962 -
6 Stirling Earl Farris Sampson, Jr. 1980 -
6 Matthew Bryan Sampson 1982 -
*2nd Husband of Karen Lynne Shuff:
+Eric Franklin Maurer 1961 -
6 Grace Sheridan Maurer 1997 -
4 John Shuff 1940 - 1940
3 Sara Pierce Matthews 1906 - 1983
+William Albert Merkel 1906 - 1984
*2nd Husband of Sara Pierce Matthews:
+Wilbur Bruns 1912 - 1993
4 Luise Bruns 1942 -
+Thomas James Zink 1935 -
*2nd Husband of Luise Bruns:
+William Frederick Thomas 1945 -
5 Sara Amelia Thomas 1971 -
+Donald F. Lebeau
*3rd Husband of Luise Bruns:
+Frederick R. Gross 1941 -
*3rd Husband of Sara Pierce Matthews:
+Melville Cochran 1913 - 1978

3 William Dunham Matthews 1907 - 1968
+Elizabeth Pechstein 1910 - 1956
4 Richard Timothy Matthews 1940 -
+Mary Sherman
5 William Matthews 1961 -
4 Elizabeth Matthews 1947 -
*2nd Wife of William Dunham Matthews:
+Mary (Dougherty) Sherman
3 Letitia Patton Matthews 1912 - 2000
+Edwin Anderson Mawhinney 1908 - 1991
4 Jere Dunham McWinn 1935 -
+Clara Jo Macon 1943 - 1978
5 Timothy Arthur McWinn 1961 -
+Elizabeth Woodford 1957 -
6 Colby Alexander McWinn 1991 -
6 Hunter Austin McWinn 1994 -
*2nd Wife of Jere Dunham McWinn:
+Genoa
5 Tabitha McWinn Abt 1981 -
5 Joshua McWinn Abt 1983 -
4 Mary Dunham Mawhinney 1942 - 1999
*2nd Husband of Letitia Patton Matthews:
+Cardinal S. Thompson 1901 - 1978
3 Stanley Matthews, Jr. 1915 - 1940
+Emily Jones
2 Lida Jere Dunham 1881 - 1950
+Elijah H. Matthews 1884 - 1929

INDEX

J

K